S0-AXP-810

Keeping Fit

A CHRISTIAN'S GUIDE TO FITNESS AND HEALTH

by Don Otis

Bible Voice Publishers
Van Nuys, California

Special thanks to

Carla Cooper Müller
for her fine job of illustrations;

Sue Forsythe Otis
for the many hours of typing;

and Winston Severn
for his expertise and assistance.

FOREWORD

As I read Don Otis' manuscript KEEPING FIT, I became enthused to think that thousands of Christians may now begin to experience what Don and I and millions of others have enjoyed for years.

We are in an age of fast-moving schedules and more conveniences than we can appreciate which require physical effort. Those conveniences need not compromise our witness of Christ by our overweight and poor health. In Ephesians, the sixth chapter, Paul talks of the Christian armor and our need to wear it — all of it — daily. We need to apply these guidelines in addressing our health needs. Exercise means to advance in better health! After all, we are charged to not "defile our temple."

Though Jesus didn't set up training guides for physical fitness or dietary programs for good food, He must have been aware of the human body's needs. In a 200-mile area which His ministry covered, He more often than not walked. maybe He occasionally rode a donkey, but the point is well made that through the rough, hilly, not climate of Palestine, He got plenty of exercise as did His disciples. So we also need to have a physically strong body that lives, breathes and exercises for Jesus Christ daily.

—Jim Ryun
World record holder
(see next page)

ABOUT JIM RYUN

For Jim Ryun, retired distance runner who set five American records and a number of world marks. The 60's saw young Ryun pile up one victory after another, including:

- Crashing the 4-minute mile barrier with a blazing 3:58.3, the fastest mile ever run by a high school athlete, May 15, 1965.
- Setting the American Citizen's record for the mile, 3:55.3, June 27, 1965.
- As an 18-year-old, bettered the 1,500-meter mark held by Dyrol Burleson of Oregon, covering the distance in 3:42.7.
- On April 23, 1966, Ryun captured the Glenn Cunningham mile in 3:55.8, a half-second slower than his own American record.
- On May 14, 1966, the 6-foot-2 runner set a new American record for the two-mile event, covering the distance in 8:25.2.
- On June 10, 1966, the 160-pounder smashed the world record for the 880, running the half-mile in 1:44.9 during the U.S. Track and Field Federation Championships.

Sets World Mile Record

- And on July 17, 1966, Ryun set the world record for the mile event at Edwards Stadium, University of California, covering the distance in 3:51.3. His time clipped 2.3 seconds off the record 3:53.6 by Michel Jaxy of France on June 9, 1965.

For his efforts, the Kansas schoolboy who trained by running 70 to 100 miles a week — was acclaimed winner of the 1966 James E. Sullivan Award as the nation's outstanding amateur athlete.

After that honor Ryun returned to the track and proceeded to:

- Break the world indoor half-mile record with a time of 1:48.3 on Feb. 23, 1967.
- Set the new world mile record of 3:51.1 on June 23, 1967, clipping two-tenths of a second off his own world mark.
- Smashed the world record for 1,500 meters with a 3:33.1 mark.

CONTENTS

Chapter One

Why Should a Christian Exercise?

"Beloved, I pray that in all respects you may prosper and be in good health, just as your soul prospers."

3 John 2

A dictionary definition of exercise says it is "bodily exertion for the sake of developing and maintaining physical fitness." The advantages of physical fitness are numerous. The physically fit body is one with a minimum of excess fat, it has good stamina and endurance for extra efforts required from work or play, and a lower cholesterol level than an unfit body. It also has an advantage of mental efficiency as well as a chance for longer life.

Not all forms of exercise lead to the physique of a Mr. Universe. Most exercises lead simply to a tightening of specific areas of the body. The result is a healthy-looking body that is strong without being "muscle-bound" (endomorphic).

Many people have a tendency toward an excess of cholesterol in their blood. Cholesterol is necessary for good health, but too much of it acts like the sludge in a carburetor of an automobile. Such sludge in the blood stream causes heart disease. Exercise helps to eliminate excess cholesterol in much the same way that fast or prolonged driving burns off carbon in an automobile engine. Just as a buildup of carbon occurs from slow and infrequent driving, so cholersterol and wastes build up in the body from easy living. Exercise cleans out the circulatory system and burns off wastes.

A study conducted at the University of Southern California showed that men between the ages of 50 and 87 exercising only three hours a week reduced nervous tension by 15%, increased oxygen consumption 9.2% and dropped diastolic blood pressure by 6%. Exercise was shown to not only increase a person's ability to relax, but indicated that people who exercised regularly had a higher performance record in their work.

Over 15 million Americans suffer some form of heart disease. Over a million die of cardiovascular illnesses. And about 750,000 people a year have heart attacks in the United States. But many physicians now require that heart attack victims exercise frequently and vigorously. The exercise not only strengthens the weakened heart but helps to build new tissues around the heart. The improved circulation improves digestion, strengthens the breathing muscles (diaphragm), improves bowel function, and increases flexibility of joints. But no one ought to wait until discovering heart disease or undergoing respiratory illness before beginning an exercise program.

The best way to increase endurance and stamina for work or play is through a regular exercise program. Many who begin to exercise discover that after a time their body begins to crave exercise. After a tiresome day at the office, the shop or in the kitchen and home, 20 or 30 minutes of running, walking, swimming or bicycling not only brings rejuvenation to a tired body, but allows for much quicker and complete rest. The exercise burns off the sense of emotional stress and fatigue, and after the exercise the body is able to rest and relax.

Another advantage of exercise, of course, is that it burns away some of those excess calories which most of us carry around as ugly fat. Obesity is not only unattractive, it is unhealthy. Fat is as much a danger to health as is disease, smoking or inactivity. Of course a certain amount of fat is necessary to keep the body insulated. But most Americans have too much of it. The reason is simple: when we consume more calories than our body is able to use, the excess calories are stored as fat. Vigorous exercise burns up some of these calories. But it takes a combination of exercise and proper diet to produce a fit body. Exercise alone is not enough. Even 100 sit-ups a day will not reduce fat around the stomach. The exercise simply tightens and strengthens the existing muscle tissue in the abdominal region. But if a proper diet is maintained, one-half hour a day of exercise can take off as much as 26 pounds of weight in a year.

It is important to keep in mind that to lose one pound of fat requires the burning of 3,500 calories. Look at the chart to see how many calories various activities require and figure out how long it would take to lose a few of those excess pounds by exercising.

Followers of Christ are referred to as temples of God in 1 Corinthians 3:16,17. "If any man defile the temple of God, him shall God destroy for the temple of God is holy, which temple ye

Activity	Speed	Calories Burned Per Hour
Bicycling	11 mph	600
Horseback riding	walk	98
Horseback riding	trot	301
Ice skating	normal	245
Jogging	11 min. a mile	648
Swimming	2 mph	553
Washing floors		84
Dishwashing		70
Ironing		70
Painting		105

are." Christ desires us to be vessels made to honor Him. Paul says in 1 Timothy 4:8, "Bodily discipline is only little profit, but godliness is profitable for all things, since it holds promise for the present life and also for the life to come." Too often we see evangelists and preachers whose lives and ministries were shortened because of needless diseases or illnesses. The body is God's marvelous creation, built with 639 muscles, 208 bones, between five and six quarts of blood and 100,000 miles of blood vessels. Each muscle fiber is about 1¼ inches long and as thick as a human hair. A muscle with a cross sectional area of one inch can lift about 140 pounds! The body is an amazing artifice. And it is made to be the temple of the living Christ.

Jesus Himself must have been an amazing man. And He serves as an example to us. He walked everywhere He went in that 200-mile area of His ministry. He worked as a carpenter before He began His ministry of teaching and healing. The rugged terrain of Palestine was His field of exercise. He fasted often. And when He did eat, He ate in moderation. He was a man who knew what He had to accomplish in the flesh, and we have every indication that He took care of His body by making it work hard. That is the secret: making the body work hard increases its ability to perform those tasks for which it was made.

Chapter Two

Vitamins and Nutrition

"Whether, then, you eat or drink or whatever you do, do all to the glory of God."
1 Corinthians 10:31

This book deals primarily with fitness, but fitness requires that some attention be given to diet and nutrition. But this book will not deal with specific diets for weight reduction, since you will find nearly all diets for weight reduction will work if they are adhered to and supplemented with proper exercise. Fluctuating weight (the so-called "fat man syndrome"), where quick weight loss is followed by quick weight gain, generally can be corrected by proper nutrition and regularized eating schedules.

Another factor which makes some attention to nutrition and diet important in an exercise book is that for good health the balance created by proper diet and proper exercise produces stamina which can maintain health when other people are succumbing to colds, flus and other contagious but minor illnesses. Moreover, it is possible to eat a perfectly balanced diet and be just the right weight and still be woefully out of condition. And the opposite situation might be the case as well: every now and then a marathon runner of note will confess to being a junk-food junky. Yet a common factor in both these cases where either improper diet or improper exercise prevail, is a susceptibility to sickness. The reason many marathon runners have an almost neurotic concern about diet is that they know how closely related diet is to physical conditioning. And for a marathon runner to catch a cold means a week of training may be lost.

But we might ask, why is it that so many Christians, including pastors, evangelists and leaders, are overweight or sick or run down? The answer seems to be that they spend little or no time taking care of their temples (their bodies). Paul says, in Romans 12:1, Christians are to be a living sacrifice: "I urge you, therefore, brethren, by the mercies of God, to present your bodies a living and holy sacrifice, acceptable [or well-pleasing] to God, which is your reasonable service of worship." One is not a living and holy sacrifice if he is tired, overweight or sick. Obesity, or overweight, for example promotes diabetes, kidney and heart problems *and* premature death. Hardly the sort of sacrifice Paul is encouraging! In the Old Testament, ceremonies of sacrifice required that only animals without spot or blemish be offered to God.

Recent conclusions reached by scientists about excess weight are startling. A person 25-35% overweight has a risk of premature death 50% above normal for any age group. Each pound of fat puts added strain on the heart and the lungs. Let's say you are 10 pounds over the life insurance chart of weights and body sizes listed below. You may look bulgy only when you peel down to your underclothes. As long as you're fully dressed you look good. Is that 10 pounds bad for you?

Here are the conclusions drawn from statistical studies: After age 45, people 10 pounds overweight will experience 8% increase in their death rate. People 20 pounds over desirable weight increase 18% their chances to die. Thirty pounds means 28% and 50 pounds means 56%.

The human body is an unfailingly accurate calorie counter. It cannot be fooled. What you put in always adds up, and if you put in more than you take out (use up), your weight goes up. If you take out more than you put in, your weight goes down. To lose weight you must eat less or exercise more, or do both.

The chart indicates proper weight according to body size, age and sex.

Breakfast

One of the simplest ways to maintain proper weight is to eat meals at regular times during the day. Make your biggest meal breakfast, not dinner. Breakfast is the most important meal. Unfortunately most people today seem to have little or no appetite in the morning. In most cases, however, a poor appetite in the morning results from eating too much the night before.

Altering the eating schedule to put more substance into breakfast does a lot to build a base of energy upon which to work a full day. Later meals don't have to be very big simply because the breakfast meal provides almost all that is needed for the day. One of the worst traps some people fall into when wanting to lose a few pounds quickly is "the fat man syndrome." That is to skip breakfast and then just snack for lunch. By 4 o'clock in the afternoon, the body cries for food substance. And since there was no breakfast

DESIRABLE WEIGHTS FOR MEN
AGES TWENTY-FIVE AND OVER

Height (with shoes, 1-in. heels)		Weight in Pounds According to Frame (as ordinarily dressed)		
Feet	Inches	Small Frame	Medium Frame	Large Frame
5	2	112-120	118-129	126-141
5	3	115-123	121-133	129-144
5	4	118-126	124-136	132-148
5	5	121-129	127-139	135-152
5	6	124-133	130-143	138-156
5	7	128-137	134-147	142-161
5	8	132-141	138-152	147-166
5	9	136-145	142-156	151-170
5	10	140-150	146-160	155-174
5	11	144-154	150-165	159-179
6	0	148-158	154-170	164-184
6	1	152-162	158-175	168-189
6	2	156-167	162-180	173-194
6	3	160-171	167-185	178-199
6	4	164-175	172-190	182-204

Source: Metropolitan Life Insurance Company. Derived previously from data of the Build and Blood Pressure Study, 1959, Society of Actuaries.

DESIRABLE WEIGHTS FOR WOMEN
AGES TWENTY-FIVE AND OVER

Height (with shoes, 2-in. heels)		Weight in Pounds According to Frame (as ordinarily dressed)		
Feet	Inches	Small Frame	Medium Frame	Large Frame
4	10	92-98	96-107	104-119
4	11	94-101	98-110	106-122
5	0	96-104	101-113	109-125
5	1	99-107	104-116	112-128
5	2	102-110	107-119	115-131
5	3	105-113	110-122	118-134
5	4	108-116	113-126	121-138
5	5	111-119	116-130	125-142
5	6	114-123	120-135	129-146
5	7	118-127	124-139	133-150
5	8	122-131	128-143	137-154
5	9	126-135	132-147	141-158
5	10	130-140	136-151	145-163
5	11	134-144	140-155	149-168
6	0	138-148	144-159	153-173

Source: Metropolitan Life Insurance Company, Derived previously from data of the Build and Blood Presure Study, 1959, Society of Actuaries.

and little lunch, the person feels justified in stuffing nearly anything and everything into his mouth to stop the hunger pangs.

If you must eat steak, pork or sausage, eat them for breakfast. Meats take the longest to digest and should be totally eliminated from the evening meal. Eggs are excellent for breakfast. They are high in protein and are good for you any way you prepare them. Fruits and fruit juices help the digestive processes and they provide carbohydrate and natural sugar for the body.

Coffee

Millions of Americans simply cannot start the day without a cup of coffee. Very few, however, are aware of the harmful effects coffee might have on both body and mind. Coffee oils irritate the stomach lining and the upper intestine. Irritating the stomach disrupts the digestive process. Coffee is also a stimulant and like other stimulants acts on the nervous system.

If you *must* have coffee, then you are addicted! If you just enjoy coffee, then substitute tea every other day, and add some milk to help neutralize the tannic acids.

Lunches

Lunch is probably the least important meal of the day. Dairy foods are especially good for you at lunchtime: yogurt, milk and cheese with a main dish consisting of fish or fowl or vegetables. Beef once in a while at noon is acceptable if it was not eaten at breakfast.

Dinner

Dinner should be the lightest meal of the day. If you limit the meal to salads, vegetables, dairy foods, juices and fish, you will sleep better and wake up feeling light and peppy. Salads are good for dinner since they assist the stomach in digestion. Keep dinner light and you will be ready for a big breakfast 10 or 12 hours later. Remember that digestion takes between 9 and 48 hours, depending on the food you eat.

Snacking

Snacks between meals should be limited to the following:

fruits	seeds
vegetables	nuts
dairy products	honey

Most weight problems occur not from eating too much, but from eating at the wrong time. If you follow the suggestions given in this chapter, and add proper exercise, your weight will drop.

Calories

What is a calorie? Few of us really know what calories are, or what they do. But we somehow conclude that calories are bad. Calories actually are measurements of heat. For each pound of body weight, a certain quantity of calories per hour are used simply for maintenance. So a calorie is a unit of measurement of how much food energy is needed to maintain a living body. In the accompanying list are a number of activities and the corresponding number of calories required to do them per pound for an hour.

The loss of one pound of body fat requires a reduction of 3,506 calories. Such a calorie loss can take place by extra exercise or by limiting food intake. You need to know what your average daily calorie requirements are. This can be discovered by figuring from the following formula:

1. A male of 154 pounds requires 2,900 calories for daily maintenance.
2. A female of 128 pounds requires 2,100 calories for daily maintenance.

For every pound you may vary from the average, add or subtract 17 calories. For example, if you are a male weighing 185 pounds, figure your caloric intake this way:

$$185 \text{ pounds}$$
$$-154 \text{ pounds}$$
$$\overline{31 \text{ pounds}}$$
$$31 \times 17 = 524 \text{ calories}$$

Adding 524 to the 2,900 required to maintain a man of 154 pounds gives a total of 3,424. A man of 185 pounds, therefore, does not need any more than 3,424 calories daily to stay at that weight. Remember, however, that the body is an un-

Activity	Calories per Pound/One Hour
Sleeping	0.43
Sitting	0.70
Housework	1.10
Walking	1.30
Jogging	1.95
Running	3.70

failingly accurate calorie counter. More than 3,-424 calories daily will mean that our 185 pound man will soon bulge with extra weight.

If you are a woman you can use the same formula, only you must be careful to use 2,100 as the base figure. And for either a man or a woman, if you weigh more than you know you ought to weigh, do the same figuring with the weight you wish you were. That will tell you how many calories you can take in a day and still lose weight. For example, if you are a man and should weigh 170 pounds, subtract 154 from 170, then multiply the difference by 17. Adding the difference to 2,900 allows you 3,172 calories a day. Sticking to a diet of 3,172 will, in time, get you down to 170 pounds.

The Basic Food Categories

Proper diet and good nutrition require foods that derive from four major groups. If diet is deficient in any one area, something will go wrong with the body. That something that goes wrong might be as minor as a problem with skin complexion or as serious as liver disease.

1. **Vegetable-fruit.** These foods provide the major quantities of vitamins and minerals necessary for health. Nearly all of the vitamin C available to humans comes out of this category. Over half of all vitamin A available through foods comes from this category. That means that growth, good vision, healthy skin, body tissue growth and maintenance require ample portions of vegetables and fruits.

2. **Meat.** Meat provides protein that is necessary for proper growth and the repair of body tissues. Muscles, blood, organs, skin and hair all require protein. From meat comes the nutrients of iron, thiamine, riboflavin and niacin.

3. **Milk.** This is the primary source of calcium needed for the growth and maintenance of bones and teeth. Milk and milk products supply various amounts of protein, riboflavin and vitamin A as well.

4. **Bread-cereals.** These supply substantial amounts of protein, iron and the B vitamins. Many fad diets call for a radical restriction or even an elimination of these foods. However, anyone who exercises strenuously will testify to the fact that the elimination of these foods can cause serious energy depletion and a susceptibility to colds, the flu and various aches and pains.

Vitamins

Many people take vitamin supplements in the form of pills or syrups. Yet few realize either the value or the danger vitamin intake might provide. Vitamins are absolutely necessary for health. Yet taken in excessive amounts, some vitamins can cause serious complications to health. The accompanying chart provides the most basic nutrients required by the body and their food sources.

Cholesterol

Cholesterol has received a lot of attention in the press and even in the advertising media recently. Cholesterol is actually a steroid that is

Nutrient	Function	Effects of a Human Deficiency	Food Sources
Carbo-hydrate	Supplies energy, aids in the function of the intestinal tract, and adds flavor to the diet	Not known	Sugars, syrups, cereal grains, legumes, and dried fruits
Fats and oils	Supplies energy and essential fatty acids, insulates the body, and protects the body organs	Not known	Vegetable oils, animal fats, and foods made with oils and fats
Protein	Builds and maintains body tissue; component of hormones, en-zymes, and antibodies; aids in the regulation of acid-base balance and osmotic pressure	Nutritional liver disease, hunger edema, pellagra, and kwashiorkor	Meats, fish, poultry, milk and its products, eggs, and nuts
Calcium	Serves as a building material for bones and teeth; necessary for the normal behavior of nerves, rhythmic beat of the heart, and clotting of blood	Tetany	Milk and its products, broccoli, citrus fruits, and leafy green vegetables (other than spinach and chard)

Phosphorus	Serves as a building material for bones and teeth, found in every cell, aids in the regulation of the acid-base balance, and necessary in muscle contraction	Not known	Meats, fish, poultry, eggs, milk and its products, and legumes
Magnesium	Involved in the use of calcium and phosphorus in the body, and an activator of certain enzymes	Gross muscular tremors	Muscle meats, nuts, vegetables, cereal grains, and milk and its products
Iron	Component of hemoglobin, the oxygen-carrying pigment of the blood	Iron-deficiency anemia	Liver, meats, egg yolk, leafy green vegetables, enriched and whole-grain cereals, and dark molasses
Iodine	Component of the thyroid hormone, thyroxine	Endemic simple goiter	Seafoods, vegetables, and iodized salt

Nutrient	Function	Effects of a Human Deficiency	Food Sources
Vitamin A	Maintains the body's epithelial tissue and serves as a component of the pigments of the eye essential for normal vision	Xerophthalmia and functional night blindness	Vitamin A: fish-liver oils, butter, enriched margarine, and egg yolk Beta carotene: yellow, yellow-red, and green fruits and vegetables
Vitamin D	Necessary for bone formation and calcium absorption and metabolism	Rickets in the young and osteomalacia in the adult	Fish-liver oils and vitamin D enriched milk
Vitamin E	Protects vitamin A and ascorbic acid from oxidation in the body	Not known	Vegetables, vegetable oils, and cereal grains
Vitamin K	Necessary for the normal clotting of blood	Hemorrhages	Cauliflower, cabbage, spinach, kale, and soybeans

Thiamine	Serves as a coenzyme in the metabolism of carbohydrates	Severe deficiency, beriberi; mild deficiency, loss of appetite, constipation, tenderness of muscle of leg calf, and mental depression	Brewer's yeast, wheat germ, pork products, legumes, and whole-grain and enriched cereals
Riboflavin	Serves as a coenzyme in the metabolism of carbohydrate, fat, and protein	Fissures in the corner of the mouth; redness of the lip membranes; greasy scaliness of the face; and in the male, scrotal dermatitis	Brewer's yeast, glandular meats, milk, cheese, eggs, leafy green vegetables, beef, veal, and salmon

Nutrient	Function	Effects of a Human Deficiency	Food Sources
Niacin	Serves as a coenzyme in the metabolism of carbohydrate, fat, and protein	Pellagra	Brewer's yeast, peanut butter, glandular meats, muscle meats, fish, and poultry
Vitamin B_6	Serves as a coenzyme in the metabolism of carbohydrate, fat, and protein	Convulsive seizures (in infants), anemia	Muscle meats, liver, vegetables, and whole-grained cereals
Folacin (folic acid)	Serves as a coenzume in the body and is necessary for normal blood formation	Anemia	Chicken livers, leafy green vegetables, and legumes
Vitamin B_{12}	Serves as a coenzyme in the body and is necessary for normal blood formation	Pernicious anemia	Liver, muscle meats, poultry, fish, and milk and its products

Ascorbic acid	Necessary in the formation and maintenance of collagen, the cementing material that holds the body cells together	Scurvy	Citrus fruits, melons, berries, tropical fruits, leafy green vegetables, broccoli, peppers, cabbages, and tomatoes
Water	Serves as a building material, a solvent, a lubricant, and a temperature regulator	First signs: weakness, weariness, thirst and dryness of the mouth	(Water), foods, beverages, and (water formed during metabolism)

present in body fluids. An overabundance of cholesterol in the system has been linked to arteriosclerosis (hardening of the arteries). Cholesterol also has been found to accumulate in the gallbladder to cause gallstones. A high intake of fatty foods can raise the level of blood cholesterol to a point where heart disease is likely.

Cholesterol is measured in milligrams and an intake of 300 milligrams or less is recommended. Limiting total fat intake to one-third of total caloric count daily and eating polyunsaturated fats rather than saturated fats can assure you of a safe level. Studies have shown that men with cholesterol levels of 265 milligrams or more in their blood have five times the chance for developing heart disease as those with blood cholesterol levels of 220 milligrams or less. A quick trip to your doctor's office for a blood test (generally administered by a nurse or a technician) can get you information about your own cholesterol count. If it is over 265 milligrams, your doctor probably will want to see you about your diet.

The main source of cholesterol is meat. Beef, pork, lamb, chicken and turkey contain between 75 and 125 milligrams of cholesterol per serving. Dairy products also contain high levels of cholesterol, although some debate has arisen concerning the amounts. When buying milk it is best to purchase low and nonfat milks. Eggs, too, are high in cholesterol. Fruits, vegetables and grains are free from ingredients which might produce blood cholesterol.

Women and Iron Deficiency

Most women do not receive sufficient iron in their diet. The recommended daily allowance (R-DA) of iron for young women is 18 milligrams. During menstruation the RDA might double or even triple. Inadequate iron in the system most commonly is indicated by excessive fatigue. Any vigorous exercise done by a woman or man suffering iron deficiency might result in physical collapse or fainting spells.

Iron is found in most meats, especially liver. Large amounts of iron are also found in dried apricots, prune juice, beans and raisins. Although non-meat foods contain some iron, the iron in meats is absorbed more easily into the system.

During menstruation women should take iron supplements if possible. There is absolutely no need to discontinue exercise because of menstruation. In fact, many women (one-third) competing in the 1976 Olympics had their menstrual periods during the competition. And many won medals. Yet, an iron supplement should be taken, particularly if a woman exercises vigorously during menstruation.

It cannot be stated often enough that proper nutrition is as important as exercise. These two, exercise and nutrition, bring to anyone both a sense of well-being and added years of service to God. If you have long neglected your body or are simply not satisfied with your appearance, then maybe it's time you changed. God, too, desires that you look and feel your best. People can learn clever ways to mask the condition of the inner man, we know. But the outward appearance is hidden to no one. The New Testament indicates that what a person is on the inside will be manifest in the outward appearance. We all know of people who never seem to be happy. In fact, they always look as though they have suffered some defeat. Yet it is the responsibility of every Christian to be an overcomer in all things. And that, of course, means the overcoming of sloth, laziness and gluttony as well as the maintenance of a prayer life, Bible study, and family time. Proper diet may be the starting place for a new life of victory for many Christians.

Chapter Three
Jogging and Running

"Do you know that those who run in a race all run, but only one receives the prize? Run in such a way that you win . . . Therefore I run in such a way, as not without aim, . . . I buffet my body and make it my slave."

1 Corinthians 9:24-27

Albert Einstein once said that human beings use between eight and 12 percent of their total brain capacity. We might modify that to say that most of us use but a small percentage of our total physical capacity. In fact, most of us exert ourselves as little as possible and think that the mark of civilization is the amount of work we do not have to do. It is true that modern technology creates many labor-saving devices, and modern civilization is defined by its technology. But one must also remember that something bad happens to the body when it becomes dependent upon the automobile rather than the legs for travel, the air conditioner rather than the sweat glands for climate control, and the artificially processed foods rather than nature for nutrition.

Modern technologically-controlled people must find ways to compensate for their artificially comfortable civilization. One important form of adjustment is special exercise. While most of us live in a world where we hardly ever have to walk any great distance or perspire for any sustained period, the body does require both. We were wonderfully and fearfully made with muscles, sinews, bones and tissues which must be extended, pulled, pushed and exerted. We *must* exercise as a special activity simply because there are so many things that are a part of modern living which keep us from doing those things that the body requires. However painful and even repugnant the thought of exercise might be for us, we *must* do it. Otherwise we risk violating the conditions of God's creation: He made us physical beings with amazing physical capabilities.

If you were to limit yourself to one form of regular exercise, jogging would probably be the best one to choose. It's true that your upper body gets very little exercise when jogging. But from a physical fitness standpoint, jogging does more for general conditioning and the prolongation of life than any other single form of exercise.

An extremely important factor in jogging is the pulse rate — the number of times your heart beats per minute (this is called a PR: pulse rate). For most men the PR is between 70 and 85. For women the range is generally from 75 to 85. An objective of exercise is to raise the PR up to 70% of its maximum. To figure your personal maximum, subtract your age from 220. An individual 40 years old should have a maximum of about 180 beats per minute. Jogging is one of the best ways to get your heart pumping that fast for a sustained period. Keep in mind that your heart needs it. The chart details age groups and percentages of maximum PR. You can find your age and see how fast you ought to get your heart beating through exercise.

If you are not accustomed to jogging, the best way to get started is a walk-run program. Begin by walking at a quick-step pace for 10 minutes. After 10 minutes, stop and check your heart rate by pressing two fingers on the inside of your arm just above the wrist. Your PR should not be as high as 70% of your maximum yet. But your heart should be beating at well above its normal PR.

The fast walk will gradually strengthen your heart muscles. Next combine walking with brief spurts of jogging. After a few weeks or a month you should be able to successfully complete the entire 10 minutes without walking at all. Having reached this point, there is virtually no limit to what you can do with jogging.

At this point you might begin to occasionally check your pulse rate while at rest. You will find that your heartbeat has actually slowed considerably. There may be actually 20 fewer beats per minute than before you started your jogging

Age Group	Max. Heart Range	80%	70%	60%	50%
18-29	203-191	162-153	142-134	119-114	101-95
30-39	190-181	152-145	133-127	113-108	95-90
40-49	180-171	144-137	126-120	107-102	90-85
50-59	170-161	136-129	119-113	101-96	85-80
60-69	160-151	128-121	112-106	95-90	80-75
70-79	150-141	120-113	105-99	89-84	75-70
80-89	140-131	112-105	98-92	83-78	70-65

program. That can total as many as 20,000 to 30,-000 fewer heartbeats a day. At the same time your lungs have become conditioned to process more air with less effort. And the number and size of blood vessels are increasing to add to the total volume of blood as much as a quart. The cardiovascular conditioning enhances muscle tone at the same time as it reduces blood pressure.

The growth of additional blood vessels improves your chances of surviving a heart attack. Any blood clot which might block proper blood circulation will stop the flow in but a small area. Normal hearts are not injured by vigorous exercise. In fact, because exercise such as jogging lowers the PR, a person can add as much as 18 days of rest per year to the heart. In the long run this might mean adding an additional year to your life over a 20-year span.

The best kind of physical fitness is "endurance" fitness. This requires keeping the heart rate high for a prolonged period of time. A high rate for an extended period affects not only the cardiovascular system but other organs and nearly all the muscles. The key to endurance exercise is oxygen intake. Everything that people do requires some energy expenditure — even sleeping. The human body produces energy by burning foods we have eaten. Almost all of us can produce enough energy to complete our daily tasks at home and work, but when it comes to more difficult or endurance jobs, few of us have enough energy. Jogging and running separates the physically fit from the physically unfit.

Every area of the body needs the benefits of oxygen. Oxygen is carried by the blood to many small and hidden areas of the body. Without proper exercise, circulation of the blood does not extend adequately to these areas. Have you ever seen a concrete wash during the summer months? Generally during the dry time of the year only small trickles of water flow down the middle. Consequently, debris accumulates on the floor of the wash. But after a strong rain, water rushes through the wash and the debris is pushed along and the floor of the wash is swept clean. Vigorous exercise affects the body in a similar way.

There are few substitutes for jogging and running, but a few are listed below in order of their effectiveness.

1. Swimming
2. Bicycling
3. Stationary running (running in place)
4. Handball
5. Basketball

You will notice that neither bowling nor weightlifting make the list. In fact, they don't even make it into the top 10 of effective exercises. This is because neither of them do for the blood system the sort of cleansing that the others do.

In the chart are various activities divided into categories by the number of beats per minute your heart will work when you do them. These are approximations and they may vary with age and physical condition.

Many fitness books list progression charts for jogging. However, since progress varies widely from person to person, I will leave the distance and times to you. A suggestion for the maintenance level would be between two- and

PULSE RATES	EXERCISES
100-110	Horseshoes, Polishing, Bicycling (5 mph), Ironing
110-120	Walking, Bowling, Softball, Archery
120-130	Golf, Exercycle, Scrubbing, Canoeing (2 mph)
130-140	Pingpong, Swimming, Climbing stairs, Shoveling
140-150	Tennis, Walking (2 mph), Badminton, Chopping wood
150-160+	Handball, Racquetball, Mountaineering, Skiing-x-country, Hockey, Running fast

three-mile runs three or four days a week. It may take up to eight weeks of jogging three times a week to reach this level. Some people enjoy daily jogs for shorter distances. But it is important to run at least three days per week. Endurance and fitness cannot be stored for very long.

Some Questions You May Have About Jogging Are Answered Below:

Q. What is the best time during the day to jog?
A. Anytime before or after the hottest time of the day. This makes early morning or late afternoon the best.
Q. Should I eat before or after jogging?
A. Always try to avoid eating before jogging. If eating is unavoidable, then wait at least one

hour, then jog. You will find that if you jog and then eat, you will not feel like eating as much as you normally might eat. So try to schedule your meals after you jog.

Q. Should I buy a warm-up suit and all the fancy trimmings now offered for joggers?

A. Actually one of the bonuses of jogging is that you need so little equipment. A good pair of shoes for running and the clothes to keep you warm when it's cold and cool are practically all it takes. Never wear plastic or rubber clothing. These prevent proper evaporation of perspiration that is necessary to maintain body temperature. Wear loose clothing that will enhance circulation of the blood.

Q. Is jogging or running any different for women than for men?

A. It is easier physiologically for women to reach a PR of 70% than it is for men. This is because women generally have smaller hearts, smaller lung capacity, and a lower hemoglobin count. Women also, incidentally, have greater resistance to pain.

Q. Is there any danger of exercising too hard?

A. There is no danger of overexercising a healthy heart. But be sure you have had your heart adequately checked before you begin a sustained program of hard exercise.

Q. Is there any way to tell if I am actually making progress in my exercise program?

A. You will soon find yourself to be sleeping better, eating better, thinking better and enjoying life more than you ever have before. And you will notice that it is easier for you to do even routine chores efficiently and with a sense of satisfaction. You may also record your distances and times on a sheet of paper. Checking PR before you start, when you return, and again 5 minutes after your return will provide you data concerning your progress.

Getting Started

Getting started is probably the most difficult aspect of jogging. Jogging is easy to read about, easy to think about, but difficult to begin doing. Often it helps to find a friend who would like to jog with you. You won't feel quite so conspicuous out on the streets and sidewalks in your shorts or sweats if someone is beside you. But oftentimes you will have to begin alone. And that requires that you find a regular time available to dress, warm up, jog and then shower. The decision to create the time indicates that you are on the way. And if you are shy about being seen shuffling along in your present physical condition, jog early in the morning or late at night.

When you begin you will experience some stiffness and soreness in your muscles and joints. That is good. If you don't feel some discomfort at first, it means you are not working hard enough. There is a big difference between pain and soreness. If you are in pain, see a doctor. If you are sore, continue to jog, because you can still jog when sore. After a time the soreness will subside. But when you first begin to jog, soreness may stay with you for as long as four weeks.

Jogging Surfaces

There are many different kinds of jogging surfaces, some of them better than others. A good surface for jogging is one that allows some give as your feet strike it. A poor surface is one that is so hard and unyielding that you can experience discomfort and pain from the ankle all the way to the lower back. In the list are various surfaces found for jogging and their relative condition.

Surface	Amount of Give	Most Prevalent
1. Sand	Good	Beaches, lakes
2. Grass	Good	Parks, Schools
3. Tarton	Above Average	Universities
4. Gravel	Fair	High Schools
5. Dirt	Fair-poor	Hills—surface
6. Asphalt	Poor	Streets
7. Concrete	Poor	Sidewalks

Generally the more give a surface has, the less pressure you put on the joints of your hips, knees and ankles. If it is difficult to find a soft surface, be sure you are jogging with a shoe that has plenty of padding. You may even want to add some additional cushioning (see Chapter 8, "Fitness Equipment"). If you have a choice, pick the softer surfaces for jogging. If you must do all or most of your jogging on the streets and sidewalks, the major injury to watch out for is the "shin splint." This is a pulling away of the muscles from the shinbone. If you begin to feel some pain in the shins after running regularly, discontinue jogging on hard surfaces for awhile. An ace bandage wrapped around the leg between the knee and the ankle will relieve some discomfort.

A helpful suggestion for jogging on streets and beaches is to measure the distance you run by driving the distance first. Record the mileage. If you do this in a few places you gain the advantage of having some variety in your workout and yet you can know exactly how many miles you are going.

Weather

Unfortunately too many people use the weather as a reason not to jog. It's a good excuse for laziness, since you can find it either too hot, too cold, rainy, snowy, slippery or threatening almost anywhere you are. Yet some of the special pleasures of jogging come when braving the cold, wind, snow, rain and hazardous terrain that inclement weather might bring. Some of the pleasure comes simply from being out there where the faint-hearted will not go. But some of the pleasure also comes from the sense of control over your own body, mind, and even the threats of nature out there. It is the thrill of overcoming.

At the same time it is not recommended that you jog during hail, sleet or driving snowstorms. Probably the most important health and safety factor in inclement weather is proper warmup before you jog. It is important to stretch the hamstring muscles (inside and back part of the upper leg) and calf muscles (behind and below the knee). Stretching prevents muscle pulls. Your muscles work much the same way as a rubber band: when it is cold the rubber becomes stiff and hard. Stretching them will prevent needless injury and soreness.

Former Olympic runner Louis Zamperini says,

"Becuase Christians believe in the soul, saved through Christ, they neglect completely the body. . . . The Scripture says, 'Why should a man die before his time?' And I think the Lord wants you to live as long as you possibly can, to serve Him as well as you can. That's why the Holy Spirit uses running as a metaphor for the ministry of a Christian. If you pace yourself properly as Paul did you will finish the course. The scripture says, 'So run.' There it is. If you take someone out of shape and put him in a race and say run to win, how can he? So running takes in more than just the day of the race. It means to train into your body those things that make you victorious."

This scripture applies not only to the spiritual, but also to the physical.

Jogging Versus Running

Why do I use the separate terms of jog and run? They are actually two different things, just like swimming using the breast stroke differs from swimming using the backstroke.

We have all seen the jogger decked out in his fancy outfit. But there are joggers of every style from sweatshirt and boxer underwear to the latest Bill Blass cashmere running suits. But while the jogger may work hard, and possibly even dress as though he were a professional, he is not yet a runner. To jog, as Webster's dictionary defines it, means to go at a slow, leisurely or monotonous pace. Running, on the other hand, is continued rapid movement. The difference is not so much in the distance covered as in the pace or speed at which it is covered. Runners are concerned about statistical data of distance and time.

Many joggers eventually do become runners because they work to improve their times over distances. The general rule is that a jogger is one who averages over 8 minutes per mile on a three mile course. You can call yourself a runner if you do it in less time.

Endurance running requires keeping a fast pace for a long period of time. Whether the distance is 220 yards or an entire marathon of 26-plus miles, pacing is a vital part of running. A good runner learns to pace himself to within several tenths of a second per quarter mile (440 yards). We can consider an example of pacing over the distance of a mile. Suppose you have been jogging two to three miles a day three or four days a week for several months and now you want to work on increasing your speed. Using an 8-minute mile we divide the mile into four segments of 440 yards (one lap around a quarter-mile track). Since we divided the distance by four, we must also divide the time by four: 8 minutes divided by 4=2 minutes. This gives an average time per lap necessary for completing a mile in 8 minutes. If you can easily do a lap in 2 minutes and then put together four 2-minute laps, you are doing a mile in 8 minutes. Then you can begin to work on going faster until eventually you do a few miles averaging less than 8 minutes per mile. When you can do that, call yourself a runner!

The Runners' Pace Chart is for those who wish to begin running.

Most major cities and some smaller towns have running events sponsored by various health-related groups or industries. The distance which seems the most popular is the 10-kilometer run

| DISTANCE | | | | | | | |
440	880	1320	Mile	1½mi	2mi	3mi	5mi
106.0	—	—	—	—	—	—	—
108.0	—	—	—	—	—	—	—
110.0	2.20	—	—	—	—	—	—
112.0	2.24	—	—	—	—	—	—
114.0	2.28	—	—	—	—	—	—
116.0	2.32	3.48	—	—	—	—	—
118.0	2.36	3.54	—	—	—	—	—
120.0	2.40	4.00	5.20	—	—	—	—
124.0	2.44	4.06	5.28	—	—	—	—
134.0	2.48	4.12	5.36	—	—	—	—
126.0	2.52	4.18	5.44	—	—	—	—
128.0	2.56	4.24	5.52	8.48	—	—	—
130.0	3.00	4.30	6.00	9.00	12.00	—	—
132.0	3.04	4.36	6.08	9.12	12.16	—	—
134.0	3.08	4.42	6.16	9.24	12.32	18.48	—
136.0	3.12	4.48	6.24	9.36	12.48	19.12	—
138.0	3.16	4.54	6.32	9.48	13.04	19.36	—

(6.21 miles). This is a good distance in which to test yourself to see if you want to be a runner. Breaking the 8-minute barrier per mile on such a run means you should hit the finish line within less than 50 minutes. If you can do that, then you are ready for a 20-kilometer run (12.4 miles) or you might even want to train for a marathon. In short, there is really no limit to what you can accomplish in running. Your only real competitor is

DISTANCE							
440	880	1320	Mile	1½mi	2mi	3mi	5mi
1.40	3.20	5.00	6.40	10.00	13.20	20.00	33.20
1.42	3.24	5.06	6.48	10.12	13.36	20.24	34.00
1.44	3.28	5.12	6.56	10.24	13.52	20.48	34.40
1.46	3.32	5.18	7.04	10.36	14.08	21.12	35.20
1.48	3.36	5.24	7.12	10.48	14.24	21.36	36.00
1.50	3.40	5.30	7.20	11.00	14.40	22.00	36.40
1.52	3.44	5.36	7.28	11.12	14.56	22.24	37.20
1.54	3.48	5.42	7.36	11.24	15.12	22.48	38.00
1.56	3.52	5.48	7.44	11.36	15.28	23.12	38.40
1.58	3.56	5.54	7.52	11.48	15.44	23.36	39.20
2.00	4.00	6.00	8.00	12.00	16.00	24.00	40.00
2.02	4.04	6.06	8.08	12.12	16.16	24.24	40.40
2.04	4.08	6.12	8.16	12.24	16.32	24.48	41.20
2.06	4.12	6.18	8.24	12.36	16.48	25.12	42.00
2.08	4.16	6.24	8.32	12.48	17.04	25.24	42.40
2.10	4.20	6.30	8.40	13.00	17.20	25.36	43.20
2.12	4.24	6.36	8.48	13.12	17.36	25.48	44.00
2.14	4.28	6.42	8.56	13.24	17.52	26.00	44.40
2.16	4.32	6.48	9.04	13.36	18.08	27.12	45.20

the clock. Your own body sets the limits. And it is a good thing to be able to say with Paul, "I have fought the good fight, I have finished the course . . ." (2 Timothy 4:7).

Chapter Four

Non-weight Exercises for Men

In this chapter I will discuss various exercises that will enhance your appearance, increase your endurance and develop greater strength. These exercises will cover the major muscle groups, beginning with the upper body and working down to the leg muscles. The charts in this chapter have been designed to help you, not to discourage you. But their effectiveness does depend upon your willingness to extend yourself to reach a particular goal.

The chest and shoulder muscles are most commonly exercised by doing *push-ups*. But there are many variations of the push-up. Diagram #1 shows the conventional push-up.

Diagram #1 Conventional push-up

With your palms shoulder length apart, facing down and with toes to the ground, keep your back straight and buttocks down. By bending *only* at the elbows, touch the tip of your nose, or your chest, to the ground. Then push your body back to the original position.

Another kind of push-up which isolates the pectoral and deltoid region for exercise is done with the use of two chairs. This is the *inclined push-up*. Space the chairs shoulder length apart and place them against a wall or a solid object.

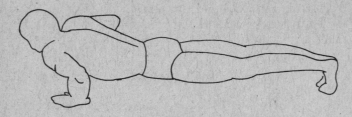

Diagram #1 Normal Push-up

Use the same motion as in the conventional push-up, letting your chest and head drop as far as possible between the chairs. The push to the starting position will be more difficult and will require more effort from the pectoral and deltoid muscles. (See Diagram #2.)

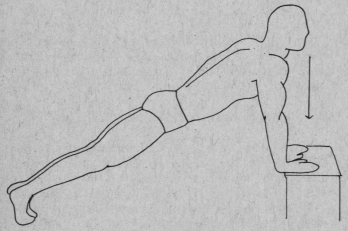

Diagram #2 Inclined push-up

Another variation is to reverse the process shown in Diagram #2 by placing your feet on the chair and your hands on the floor. This is the *decline push-up* and even more difficult to do. But it strengthens the shoulder, back, and chest areas by putting more weight on those muscles.

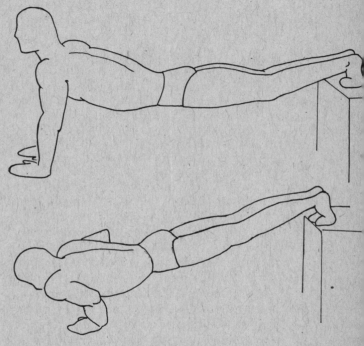

Diagrams #3 & 4 Decline push-up

When doing push-ups try to keep the body in a straight line. Avoid bending the body in any way. Keep the stomach pulled in, the arms straight, and the head and neck following in a line from the back. To make the push-up slightly more difficult, try spreading your palms past your shoulders.

PUSH-UPS (CONVENTIONAL)

AGE	End of Week 2	Week 4	Week 6	Week 8 (maintenance level)
18-29	20-25	25-30	30-35	35-45
30-39	15-20	20-25	25-30	30-40
40-49	10-15	15-20	20-25	25-35
50-59	5-10	10-15	15-20	20-30
60-69	0-5	5-10	10-15	15-25

The Push-Ups progression chart is broken down into two-week phases. Follow the suggested workout schedule at the end of this chapter and you will find yourself with an increased strength in the chest and shoulders within only two or three weeks.

The next exercise good for developing the shoulders and the arms is *the dip*. This exercise is done using two chairs. Place the chairs with the backs facing one another. Place your hands on the top of each chair back. Start with your elbows in a locked or straight position. Bend your legs at the knees so that your feet are off the ground and your body weight is resting on your extended arms. Then dip your body between the chairs, bending your arms at the elbows. Then push your body back to a locked arm position. Repeat. (See Diagram #5.)

A good alternative exercise is the *pull-up* or chinup. Few people find the pull-up an easy or fun exercise. If you are able to do one pull-up, that is a good start. Many men have difficulty doing even one. But don't be discouraged if you

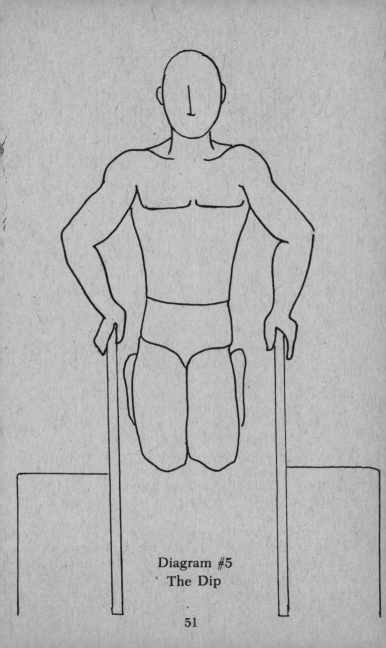

Diagram #5
The Dip

51

can't. Begin by simply hanging from the bar as long as you can. This strengthens the forearms, shoulders and upper back muscles until eventually they are strong enough to pull the body upward toward the bar.

You will need a strong iron bar or a pull-up bar. Pull-up bars are found at most grade schools

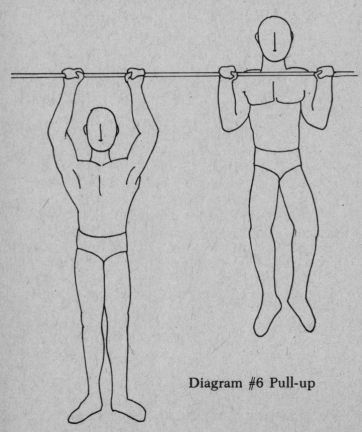

Diagram #6 Pull-up

and colleges. Or you can buy one at a sporting goods store that will fit into any normal door frame in your home or apartment. To begin the pull-up, grasp the bar overhand, then pull your body up until your chin is above the bar. (See Diagram #6.)

PULL-UPS (CONVENTIONAL)

AGE	End of Week 2	Week 4	Week 6	Week 8 (maintenance level)
18-29	4-7	6-9	8-11	10-13
30-39	3-6	5-8	7-10	9-12
40-49	2-5	4-7	6-9	8+
50-59	1-4	3-6	5-8	7+
60-69	0-3	2-5	4-7	6+

An alternative to the pull-up is to bring the back of your neck to the bar instead of your chin. This is a difficult exercise and may take some time to master, since muscles not normally used need to be developed. But it is a good exercise for the upper back, the shoulders, and the triceps.

Another alternative exercise for the triceps is the *tricep lever*. Place two chairs shoulder distance apart against a solid object. Put your palms on the edge of the seat of each chair, with your buttocks between the chairs and your legs straight out, heels to the ground. Now bend the elbows and let your buttocks drop as far as possible. Then return to the original position. (See Diagram #7.)

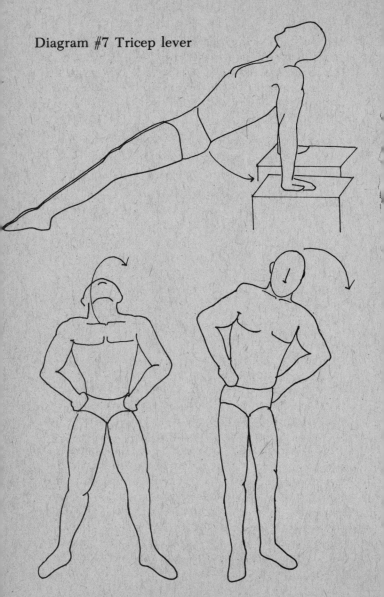

Diagram #7 Tricep lever

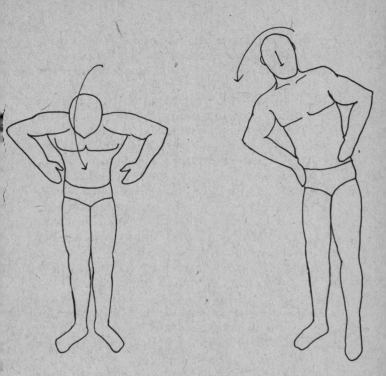

Diagrams #8, 9, 10 & 11 Trunk twisters

Several less strenuous exercises used for loosening up the lower back muscles and waist are *trunk twisters*. The trunk twister is done starting with hands on hips and legs spread slightly apart. The first movement is to bring your head forward and down past your waist. The second movement is to the right, then backward, then to the left and up again. Sound complicated? It is really simple to do. Follow these diagrams to get started. (See Diagram #8, 9, 10 and 11.)

A variation of the full trunk twister is an exercise we might simply call the *twister*. Stand erect with hands clasped behind the neck. On the first count, bend forward so that your back is nearly parallel to the floor. Remain in that position. Then touch your left elbow to your right knee while keeping your legs locked in place at the knee. Then touch your right elbow to your left knee and return to an upright position.

To increase forearm and wrist strength, do the *wrist curl*. The help of a metal bar or a broom handle is all you will need to do this exercise. Hold the bar in both hands, palms down and arms straight in front of you. Simply twist the bar in a circle. If this movement is too easy, attach a strong string about 3 feet long and a weighted object to the string. Then roll the bar and lift the object.

The following exercise for the mid and lower back region is called the *hip raiser*. Lie flat on your back, legs straight. Keep your arms at your side, lift your buttocks and hips off the floor. Hold that position for 5 to 10 seconds. Then return to the first position. Remember to keep your shoulders on the floor. (See Diagrams #12 & 13.)

After you feel you have mastered the hip raiser as described above, try folding your hands on your chest. This will make the exercise slightly more difficult.

The previous set of exercises are designed to strengthen the upper body muscles. But another area is probably in equal need for exercise. That is the abdominal region.

But before looking at various exercises for the abdomen it is important to note that exercises such as *sit-ups, leg raisers* and various *dips* and *bends* will not necessarily take off weight. Exercises tighten and firm existing tissue. Some people can and will lose weight around the waist by doing these exercises. But the primary benefit is to tighten the muscles and fat tissue. You will not lose a substantial amount of weight doing sit-ups, or any other exercise.

Probably the best known exercise for the stomach is the *sit-up*. However, like the push-up there are many variations. You should begin with the conventional sit-up. Have a friend or spouse hold your ankles. If no one is available to help, use the edge of a bed or a heavy chair. Bend your knees and lie back on the floor. Fold your hands behind your neck, then sit up and touch your elbows to your knees. (See Diagram #14.)

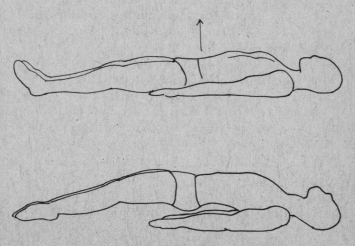

Diagrams #12 & 13 Hip raiser

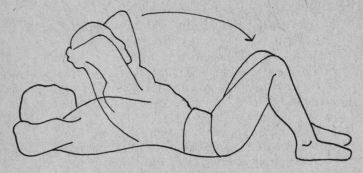

Diagram #14 Sit-up

Variation 1. Follow the same procedure as explained in Diagram #10, except this time place your hands in a folded position on your chest. This forces you to use only your abdominal muscles.

Variation 2. Using a chair or bench, sit and drop your body backwards until your head touches the floor. Then return to a sitting position. (See Diagram #15.)

SIT-UPS: 60 SECONDS
PROGRESSION CHART

AGE	End of Week 2	Week 4	Week 6	Week 8 (maintenance level)
18-29	35-40	40-45	45-50	50-55
30-39	30-35	35-40	40-45	45-50
40-49	25-30	30-35	35-40	40-45
50-59	20-25	25-30	30-35	35-40
60-69	15-20	20-25	25-30	30-35

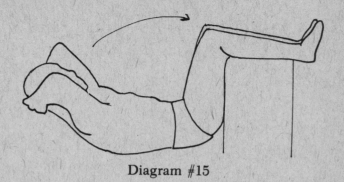

Diagram #15

Variation 3. Touch your right elbow to your left knee, then your left elbow to your right knee. This works the waist muscles as well as the abdominal muscles.

Another exercise for the stomach area is the 4-count *leg raiser*. Lie flat on your back, legs straight and arms at your sides. Lift your legs 12 inches off the floor, keeping your ankles together. Then spread your legs as wide as possible. Bring them back together and then down. Repeat. (See Diagram #16, 17 and 18.)

A variation of the leg raiser is to bring your knees to your chest. Then straighten your legs without letting them touch the floor. (See Diagram #19.)

If you have access to a bench, the following abdominal, waist, and lower back exercise is good. Lie flat on your stomach with your upper torso hanging off one edge. (You will need someone or something to hold your legs to the bench.) With your hands folded behind your neck, drop your upper body to the floor until your head touches the floor. Then return to a parallel position. (See Diagram #20)

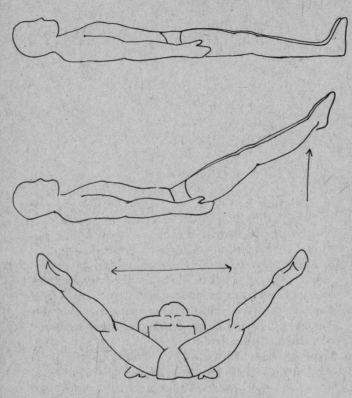

Diagrams #16, 17 & 19 Leg raiser

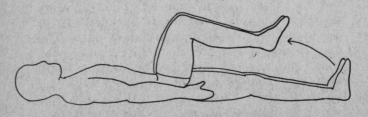

Diagram #19 Variation leg raiser

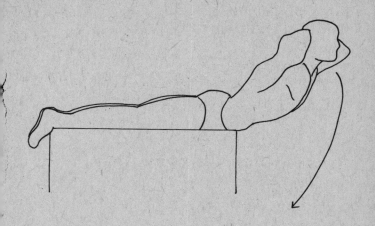

Diagram #20 Back arch

You may experience some lower back pain at first while doing the abdominal exercises. If you have a weak back and the pain persists, stick with the conventional sit-up until your back muscles become stronger.

A lot of attention has been devoted recently to the development of the leg muscles, with all kinds of running and jogging books being published. A good way to develop strength in the legs for even more effective jogging is to exercise the thighs and the calf muscles. The thighs are the upper part of the leg (above the knee). There are several good exercises for the thighs. The *knee bends* are a starter. Set a chair behind you, stand straight and extend your arms in front, keeping your back straight. Sit slowly until your buttocks lightly touch the chair, then return to a standing position. Do not use the chair to rest! (See Diagram #21.)

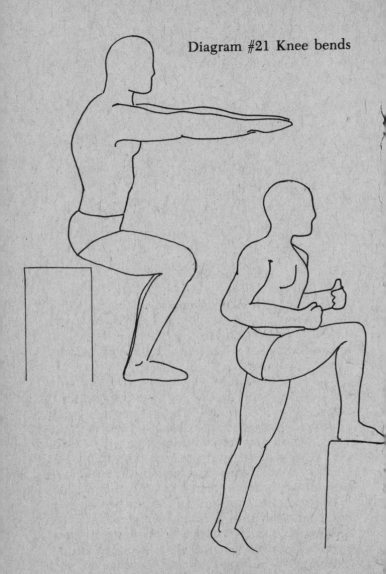

Diagram #21 Knee bends

Diagram #22 Step-up

Another very good exercise for the thighs is called the *step-up*. As the name implies, it is done simply by stepping up onto an object 16 to 18 inches high. You may use a bench or sturdy chair. Or you might use the second step in a staircase. (See Diagram #22.)

An alternative exercise for the thighs is called the *mountain-climber*. Start in a push-up position, legs extended, and body weight resting on your arms. Bring your right leg forward with your knee under your chest, then return it to the extended position. Repeat the same process with the left leg. (See Diagram #23.)

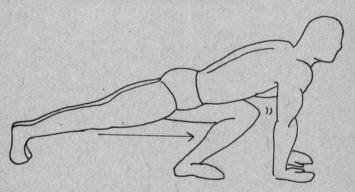

Diagram #23 Mountain-climber

The calf muscles are located directly below the knee, behind the shinbone. An excellent warm-up exercise using the calf muscle is the *jumping jack*. Stand straight, hands at your sides, ankles together. In one quick motion touch your palms together above your head, keeping elbows straight. Simultaneously spread your legs apart in a short jump. Then return back to the standing position with hands at your sides. Jump as rapidly as possible this way for as many as 30 repetitions. (See Diagram #24.)

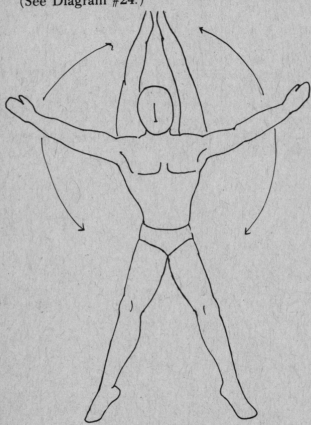

Diagram #24 Jumping jack

Now that your legs are loose, find a brick or the edge of a stair for an exercise called the *toe raiser*. Stand with your toes to the end, heels hanging over the edge. Then dip down as far as you can go and then extend back up on your tiptoes. You should be able to do at least two sets of 25. (See Diagram #25.)

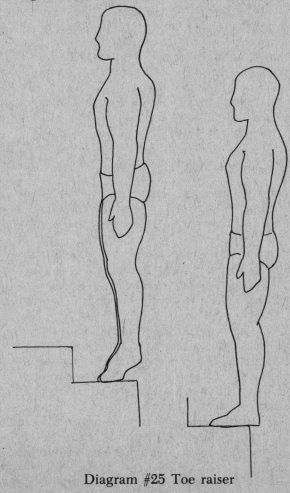

Diagram #25 Toe raiser

The further you can extend your heels below the level of your toes, the more effective the conditioning for the calf muscles is.

Some people will find these exercises difficult at first. But the longer a person stays with a program of exercise, the more routine it all becomes. Do not be discouraged if you find yourself struggling with the exercises at first. You are not competing against anyone but yourself. You may find it more relaxing and somewhat easier to exercise with a group of friends from your church. Or another way to make the session more enjoyable is to exercise while watching a ballgame on television or a newscast. Or you may listen to music which provides a background rhythm.

These exercises are especially valuable for those people who find themselves traveling a good deal. All of the above exercises can be done comfortably in a hotel room. And if a travel schedule has in the past given you an excuse not to exercise, after reading this chapter, the excuse doesn't work anymore. But the best thing is that you will feel better, you will work better, and you will serve God better.

The charted programs that follow are designed to help you get started on a three-day-a-week program. After a short while you may want to increase your exercise program to four or five days a week. These charts serve as suggestions and you may wish to insert your own variations to some exercises. But the charts cover all major muscle groups. And if you substitute or change an exercise, be careful not to eliminate any important muscles.

Finish your chest workout with the following

loosening up exercise called *chain breakers*. Stand straight with your legs slightly spread and bring your hands together at the chest, elbows up. Throw your elbows back, as if you were stretching a large rubber band. Repeat this 10 to 12 times. (See Diagram #26.)

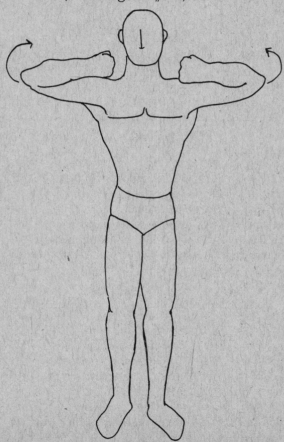

Diagram #26 Chain breakers

DAY 1 CHEST, SHOULDERS, BACK

Exercise	Sets	Repetitions	Muscles
1. Jumping jacks	1	25-30	Warm-up
2. Push-ups	2	See Chart	Chest-Shoulder
3. Incline Push-ups	2	Maximum	Upper Chest-Shoulders
4. Decline Push-ups	2	Maximum	Lower Chest-Shoulders
5. Dips	2	Maximum	Shoulders-Back

DAY 2 ARMS

Exercise	Sets	Repetitions	Muscles
1. Pull-ups	2	See Chart	Back, Shoulders, Forearms, Biceps
2. Push-ups (Hands out)	2	Maximum	Shoulders, Triceps
3. Tricep lever	2	Maximum	Back of Triceps
4. Wrist curl	2	10-15	Forearms, Wrists
5. Jumping jacks	1	25-35	Warm Down

DAY 3 STOMACH AND LEGS

Exercise	Sets	Repetitions	Muscles
1. Jumping jacks	1	25	Calves, Warm-up
2. Sit-ups	2	15-20	Stomach
3. Toe raisers	2	15-20	Calves
4. Leg raisers	2	8-12	Stomach
5. Squats or Step-up	2	8-12	Thighs

There are substitutions you can make for several of the exercises listed above. For example, you may want to do sit-ups on an inclined board so that your feet are above your head when you lie down. Or instead of squats you may do either the mountain-climber or the step-up. If you have a weak or frequently sore lower back, incorporate the hip-raiser into any of the three workouts.

But remember that the most difficult exercise of all is not that of the body but of the mind. Even as you become more proficient in a given field by exercising discipline, so also you can become more proficient in exercise of the body by discipline. How often have you heard a friend say, "I really didn't feel like praying or reading my Bible today?" But then he will say, "God gave me a real breakthrough in prayer," or "God opened up the scriptures to me in a special way," after he went ahead and read and prayed in spite of his feelings. The same principle of discipline works with exercise. No one is going to make you do it. God grants us freedom of choice. And choices inevitably produce consequences. Your choices about exercise are directly related to consequences that have to do with a temple prepared or unprepared for the King. "Do you not know that you are a temple (sanctuary) of God, and that the Spirit of God dwells in you?" (1 Corinthians 3:16).

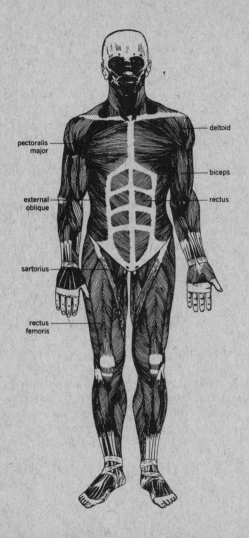

deltoid

pectoralis major

biceps

external oblique

rectus

sartorius

rectus femoris

MUSCLES OF THE HUMAN BODY. This drawing shows, front and back, the layer of muscles directly under the skin. Only a few of these muscles, the largest and most familiar, have been labeled. There are many other muscles underneath this top layer. It would require a great number of drawings to show all the muscles of the human body.

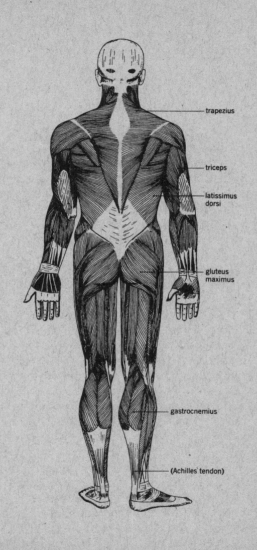

trapezius

triceps

latissimus
dorsi

gluteus
maximus

gastrocnemius

(Achilles tendon)

Chapter Five

Weight Lifting for Men

Lifting weights can be more than just a body building experience. Weight lifting is as much a sport and a challenge as playing tennis, golf or running a marathon race. The primary difference is that the individual competes only against himself. The only opponent is the weight being lifted. The good thing about this is that the weight cannot cheat or do anything clever. Therefore the weight lifter always knows the score.

There is no specific amount of weight that any person should be able to lift. Age and body size do not really matter as much as many people suppose they do. Many men with relatively small body size can lift a great amount of weight after training carefully.

The illustrations on pages 70-71 show some of the muscles that I will talk about in this chapter. I will diagram exercises which will help improve each of them.

The chest muscles known as the *pectoralis major* are what many people want strengthened by weight lifting. The exercise used often for enlarging and strengthening the pectorals is the *bench press*. (See Diagram #1.)

This exercise is done using a padded bench with two standards at one end to hold the barbells. Enough weight should be put on the bar

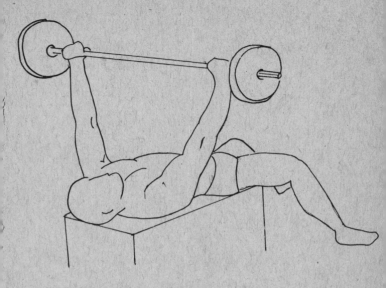

Diagram #1 Bench press

to be able to do at least 8 repetitions but not more than 12. Take a supine position on the bench, raise the bar off the standards, lower it to your chest and then press it upward.

You will experience some soreness after bench pressing. But the body soon adjusts and you will gradually find yourself increasing the weight.

Another good exercise for the chest is the *inclined press*. This requires a bench that adjusts so that the back can rest on an inclined plane. The inclined bench press can be done with either dumbbells or the barbells.

A third chest exercise, done with dumbbells, is the *flat bench press*. First, pick up the weights, keeping your seat on the bench and raise the dumbbells to your chest. Then lean back and

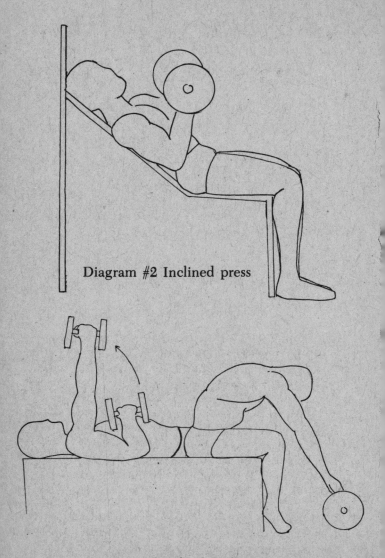

Diagram #2 Inclined press

Diagram #3 Flat bench press

push the dumbbells straight out from your chest. (See Diagram #3.) Bring your arms together so that the weights touch together above your chest.

A variation of this is the *decline press*. Just like the flat bench press, the decline press is done using dumbbells. They are raised above the chest, touched together, and brought back down to the chest.

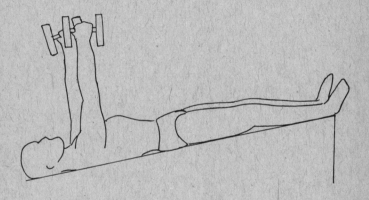

Diagram #4 Decline press

Another large group of muscles found near the top of the back and below the neck are the *trapezius*. The best exercise for this group is called *rowing*. Rowing can be done in a variety of ways. The barbells seem to work the best, however. Stoop down and lift the barbell to your waist (see Diagrams 5, 6 & 7), arms straight and hands close together on the bar. Pull the bar to your chin and then let it back down to your waist. Repeat the motion.

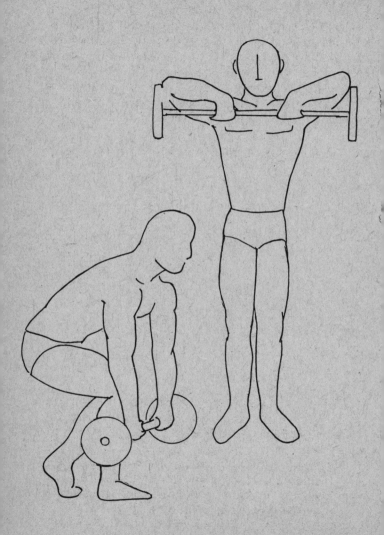

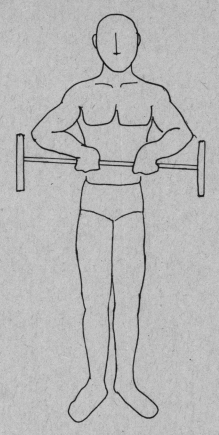

Diagrams #5, 6 & 7 Rowing

The top of the shoulders can be strengthened also by doing *upright flys*. These are done with dumbbells. Place your hands on the weights, palms in, elbows straight. Bring the weights above your head and touch them together. (See diagrams 8 and 9.)

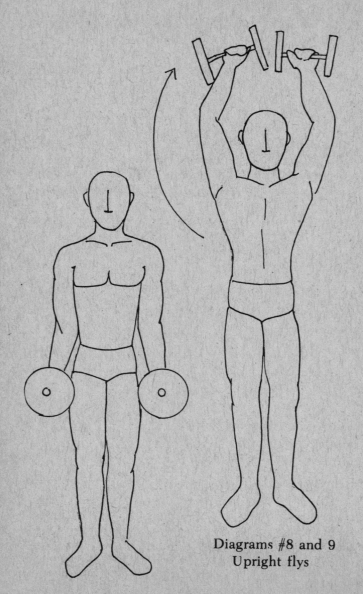

Diagrams #8 and 9
Upright flys

The *deltoids* are the muscles located just in the front of the shoulders. These muscles are partially exercised when doing any chest exercise. One of the direct exercises for the deltoids is called *supine flying*. Lying on your back on a flat bench, take a light dumbbell in each hand. Without bending the elbow, drop your arms as far as possible and bring the weight directly above your head. You will find it necessary to use a weight lighter than in the previous exercises. With supine flying and the other dumbbell exercises it may take several workouts before you feel comfortable and stable with the weight in your hands. Don't stop just because the weights feel awkward. (See diagram #10.)

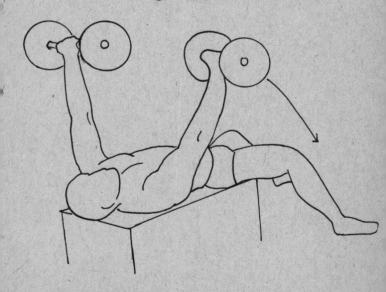

Diagram #10 Supine flying

79

Between the shoulder and the elbow are the leverage muscles, called the *biceps* and the *triceps*. The biceps are on the front of the arm and the triceps in the back. There are many exercises effective for building and maintaining these muscles. The most widely known exercise is the

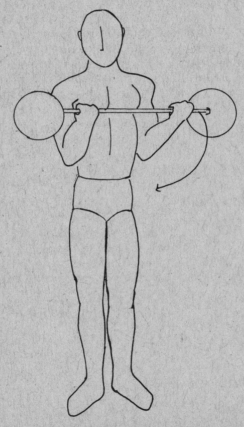

Diagram #11 Curl

curl. This can be done either standing or sitting with dumbbells or with barbells. Using a barbell in a standing position, start by picking up the weight, palms out. Stand with your back straight (up against a wall preferably) and bring the bar to your chest by bending at the elbow and pulling upward with your forearms. (See Diagram #11.)

For more isolated work on the biceps, bring the bar up only to the point that your wrists and forearms are parallel to the floor. Hold and then repeat the motion. This is more difficult because it exhausts the muscles rapidly, giving them little or no rest between repetitions.

To strengthen the forearms at the same time do the *reverse curl.* Grip the bar overhand, palms down. Then use the same motion as in the conventional curl.

You can perform virtually the same exercise with dumbbells. As you lift with one arm, keep the other at your side. (See Diagram #12.)

The triceps are best exercised by an over-the-head lift called the *tricep extension.* With the assistance of a bench, lie down flat with your head on the bench. Place the weight on your chest, gripping one end of the dumbbell. Lift the weight up from your chest, extending your arms upward. (See Diagram #13.)

An easy variation to the previous exercise is to extend the weight behind your head reaching backwards toward the ground. This exercise can be done with a barbell also.

The *reverse military press* is good for the triceps as well as for the upper and lower back muscles and shoulders. This is done either standing or sitting. The trick is to place the weight

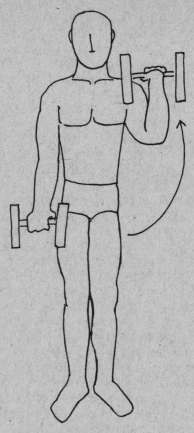

Diagram #12 Reverse curl

behind your neck. A bench with standards for the bar is helpful. Place the barbell or dumbbells behind your head so that the weight rests on your shoulders. Press the bar above your head. (See Diagrams #15 and 16.)

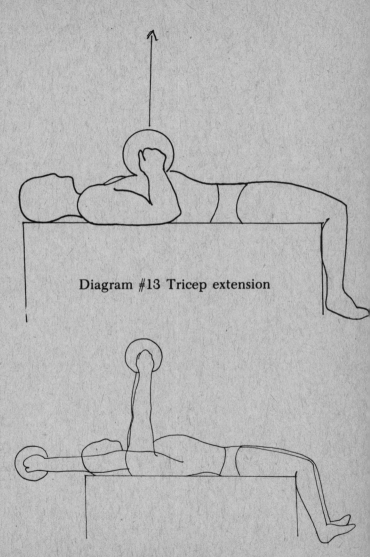

Diagram #13 Tricep extension

Diagram #14 Variation of tricep extension

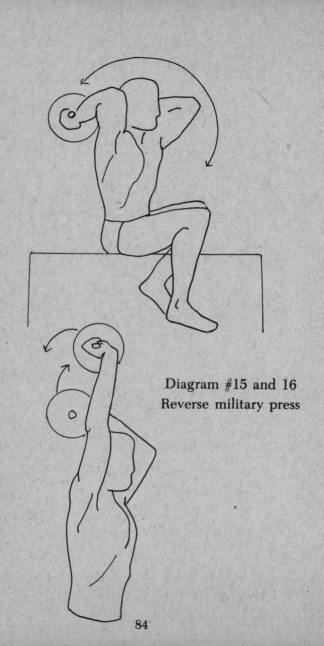

Diagram #15 and 16
Reverse military press

A less talked about muscle in the arm is what is called the *extensor digitorum profundus*. You know it as your forearm. It is used for everything from writing to driving. One of the advantages of using dumbbells for exercise is that the forearm gets a lot of work in every exercise you do. Simply to hold a dumbbell exercises the forearm muscle.

But if you want to add bulk or strength to your forearm, try the *wrist curl*. Set a barbell with very little weight. Find a strong surface over which you can lean your forearms. Use short, quick wrist movements with your palms in or out, depending on which side of the forearm you wish to develop. (See Diagrams #17 & 18.)

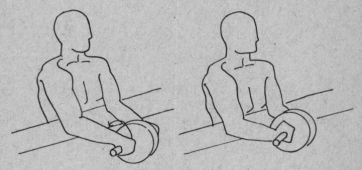

Diagrams #17 & 18 Using a counter

Continue the movement until you feel a burning sensation in the forearm and wrist region. This should take about 20 to 25 repetitions.

To this point I have covered the most important muscles of the upper body. Now I will discuss the leg muscles. The muscle you should be using the most when doing any kind of lifting is called the *rectus femoris*. This is located between the waist and the knee. The muscle is commonly referred to as the thigh. A large percentage of backaches are caused by improper lifting of heavy objects. An improper lift can put as much as 3,000 to 5,000 pounds per square inch on the lumbar discs of the spine. A rule always to follow when lifting is "Bend your knees, not your back!"

The best exercise for the thigh muscles is the *knee bends* or the *squat*. Place a barbell across the back of your shoulders with your palms facing out. Then slowly sit down until your buttocks graze a bench or chair positioned behind you. Keep the tension on the thighs by not actually sitting. (See Diagram #19.)

Make sure that you use a chair or a bench behind you. Otherwise you will probably go too far down. And squatting too far can cause severe knee damage.

Invariably you will experience shaky legs after your first few workouts. This does not mean that you are hurting the muscles. Continue with your regular workout schedule. The shaky feeling means you are doing some good to your leg muscles.

Below the knee and extending down to the ankle is the *gastrocnemuis*, the calf muscle. The front of the calf, to the right of the shinbone, is a muscle rarely exercised except while walking. A simple, yet effective exercise for this muscle is the *reverse toe raiser*. Place a dumbbell or barbell on the floor in front of you, put one of your feet under the weight, and lift it. You can lift it by rocking back on your heels. (See Diagram #20.)

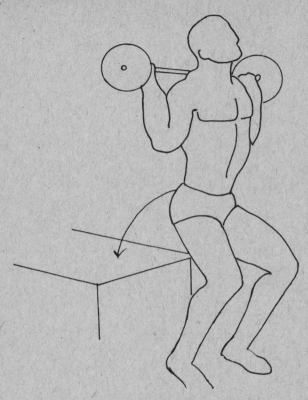

Diagram #19 Knee bends or squats

An excellent exercise for the back of the calf is the regular *toe raiser.* (See Diagram #21.) This is done with the use of a stair or anything else that you can stand upon. Stand on the object so that your heels lean over the edge. Place a light barbell on the back of your shoulders, holding the bar palms out. Stand so that your toes and the balls of your feet are securely on the edge. Then

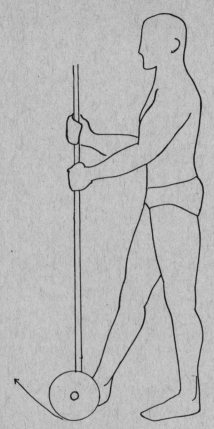

Diagram #20 Reverse toe raiser

rise to your toes, then back down. You should use a weight that will allow you to complete at least 12 — 15 repetitions. This exercise will cause a burning sensation in the muscles.

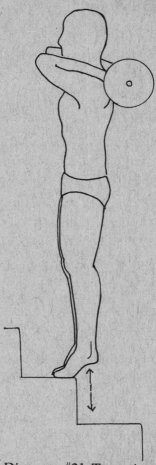

Diagram #21 Toe raiser

The two previous exercises not only strengthen the legs but the ankles also. Strong ankles and legs are essential for many sports such as tennis, cycling, swimming, jogging and racketball.

For nearly all of the exercises mentioned so far, there are good variations. You may even find that you like one of your own variations better than one of these. But these exercises are reliable for building and maintaining muscle, bulk, stamina and appearance.

When lifting weights it is important to remember that soreness is inevitable for the beginner. Keep up your workouts despite minor muscle soreness. To avoid serious muscle strains or pulls be sure to warm up prior to a workout. There will be times when you are in a hurry or just want to get the workout finished. But be careful not to neglect warming your muscles before doing heavy lifting.

Because muscles begin to deteriorate 72 hours after a workout, it is a good idea to work out at least three days a week. Each workout should last a minimum of 30 minutes. If you don't have at least that much time, don't even bother to begin a workout — do it the next day.

During a workout it is important to exhaust the muscle used for each exercise. This means that you should be so tired on the last repetition that you can barely lift the weight to perform the exercise.

Next I want to present a practical workout pattern. Since there are two types of muscles, *flexors* and *extensors*, it is best to concentrate on one set or the other during a particular workout. Flexors are the muscles that assist a joint in bending or flexing. Extensors are the muscles which extend a bodily part. An example of an extensor is the tricep muscle. The following charts give ideas about getting started with weight lifting exercises.

DAY 1 CHEST AND BACK

Exercise	Sets	Repetitions	Weight Type
1. Bench press	3	8-12	Barbell
2. Incline press	3	8-12	Barbell
3. Rowing	3	8-12	Barbell
4. Upright flys	3	8-12	Dumbbell
5. Supine flys	3	8-12	Dumbbell

DAY 3 ARMS

Exercise	Sets	Repetitions	Weight Type
1. Curls (standing)	3	8-12	Dumbbell-Barbell
2. Tricep extension	3	8-12	Dumbbell
3. Wrist curl	3	15-18	Barbell
4. Reverse military	3	8-12	Barbell
5. Tricep extension, Variation 1		8-12	Dumbbell-Barbell

DAY 5 LEGS

Exercise	Sets	Repetitions	Weight Type
1. Toe raisers	3	15-18	Barbell
2. Reverse toe raiser	3	15-18	Barbell-Dumbbell
3. Squats	3	15-18	Barbell

The charted routine covers the major muscles during a week's time. Be sure that you set your weights properly and secure them with the collars provided.

If you wish to work primarily on endurance, decrease the weights and increase the amount of repetitions to 12–15 on each exercise. If on the other hand you wish to increase muscle tone and/or weight, you should decrease the repetitions to 6–8 an exercise. An increase in weight on the bar should correspond to the decrease in repetitions.

A disadvantage of bulkiness is that it hampers flexibility. An advantage is that a bulky person usually has additional strength. Depending on your personal interests you can either increase or decrease the size of your body by what you do with weight and repetitions. But the three-day-a-week pattern of exercises should be maintained, using Monday, Wednesday, Friday sequence or a Tuesday, Thursday, Saturday sequence.

Another important aspect of weight training is proper breathing. Proper inhaling and exhaling can increase your strength and repetition number. Proper breathing helps also to circulate the flow of oxygen through the system. An example of proper breathing can be illustrated by the bench press. The air should be exhaled while the bar is pressed upward from your chest. Air should be inhaled when the weight is brought back down to the chest. The chest cavity will hold the unreleased air if it is not allowed to escape. And that builds a good deal of pressure in the chest and concomitantly increases blood pressure. If you have any circulatory weakness at all, improper breathing or holding the breath during weight training exercises could be hazardous. Above all, do not hold the breath while lifting.

Chapter Six

Weight and Non-weight Exercises for Women

Part 1

A false notion about weight training for women is that it causes bulk. Most women don't want to be looked upon as muscle-bound. But as we saw in the last chapter, weight training does not necessarily create bulk. Light weights, coupled with many repetitions, create long, sinewy muscles.

All of the exercises in this chapter are to be done with dumbbells. Lifting these weights at first will feel awkward. One dumbbell may feel heavier than the other or you may feel unbalanced when holding them. But after a short while you will become accustomed to holding weights in your hands, and the exercises will seem easy.

The exercises which follow will concentrate on one exercise for each muscle group and then one alternate exercise for each group. The alternative example of an exercise is given simply for variety in the program. You may substitute exercises of your own so long as they relate to the muscles under consideration.

Exercise #1: *Standing Flys* (See Diagram 1.)
Muscles: shoulders, arms

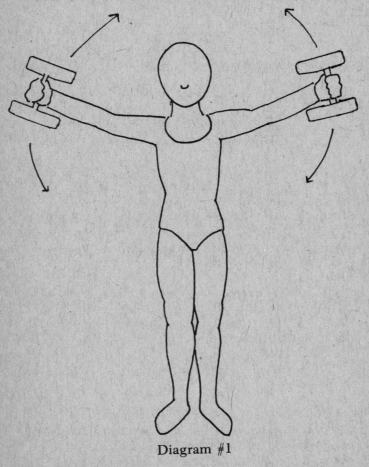

Diagram #1

Movement. Hold a very small dumbbell in either
hand and extend your arms so that the elbows are

straight. Keep your elbows locked straight, lift the weights above your head and touch them gently together over your head. Then bring them down to your hips. Repeat the movement.

Alternative exercise: *Bent-over Lateral Rise*
Muscles: shoulders, upper back (See Diagram 2.)

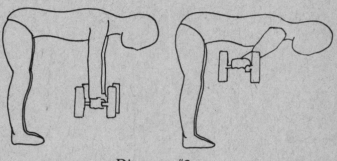

Diagram #2

Movement. Bend over at the waist with your arms straight toward the floor. Using a light weight, straighten your arms so that they are even with your back. Then return to the starting position.

Exercise #2: Bent-over Rowing (See Diagram #3.)
Muscles: upper back, chest, forearms

Movement. Bend forward at the waist, holding the weights in front of you, arms straight. Using one arm, bring the dumbbell to your chest, straighten your elbow. Then repeat the movement with the opposite arm.

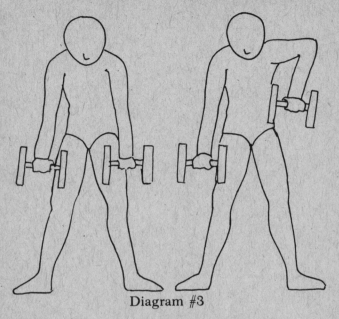

Diagram #3

Alternative exercise: *Upright Rowing* (See Diagrams #4 & 5)

Muscles: upper back, shoulders, forearms

Movement. Stand straight, legs slightly spread. Bring the weights to your chest simultaneously, bending your elbows. Then straighten the elbows again with the weights at the top of your thighs. Repeat the same motion for one repetition.

Exercise #3: *Modified Bench Press* (See Diagram #6.) Muscles: chest, shoulders

Movement. Lying flat on a bench extend your arms straight above your chest until the dumbbells are at arms' length. Lower them to the sides of your chest, then push them back to the extended position.

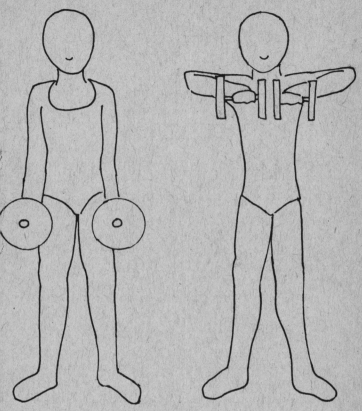

Diagrams #4 & 5

Alternative exercise: *Forward Arm Lift* (See Diagram #7.) Muscles: chest, shoulders, arms

Movement. Start with your legs spread shoulder width, gripping the dumbbells in both hands (palms in). Stand straight and lift the weights directly in front of you. The motion is actually a half circle from your hips to straight in front of

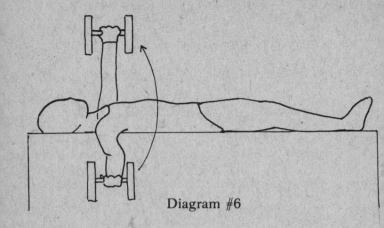

Diagram #6

your chest. Either of the two exercises just
described are excellent for increasing or tightening the bust area.

Exercise #4: *Bent Arm Pull-overs* (See Diagram
#8.)
Muscles: back of the arms (triceps) and chest

Movement. Stand straight with feet spread
shoulder width. Hold one dumbbell over the
head and lower the weight slowly behind your
neck by bending your elbows. Pull back up again
and repeat.

Alternate exercise: *Supine Pull-over* (See
Diagrams #9 & 10.)
Muscles: triceps, chest

Movement. Lie flat on a bench, weight extended
over your head. Holding the dumbbell at one
end, extend it as far toward the floor over your
head as possible.

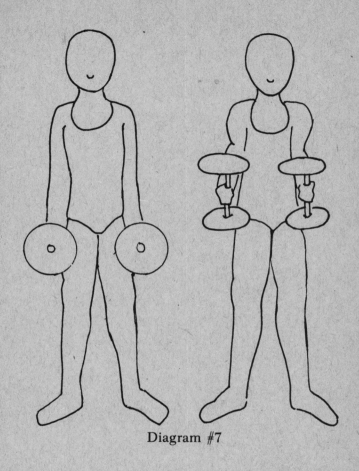

Diagram #7

Exercise #5: *Standing Curls* (See Diagram #11.)
Muscles: front of arms (biceps)

Movement. Hold a dumbbell in each hand. With
your arms dropped to below your waist, lift the
dumbbell to your chest, bending your arms at the
elbows. Your elbows should be tucked into your

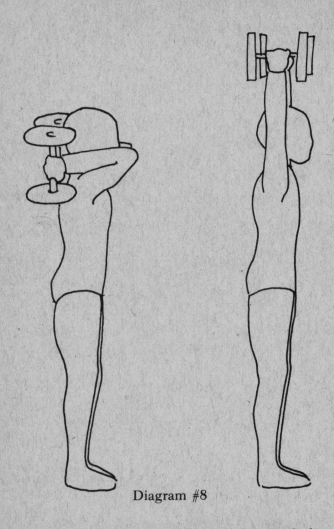

Diagram #8

sides as you lift the weights. Be sure to pick the dumbbell up so that your palms are facing outward from your body.

100

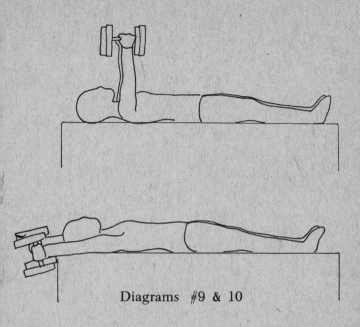

Diagrams #9 & 10

Alternative exercise: *Isolated Curls* (See Diagram #12.)
Muscles: biceps, forearms

Movement. Set your elbows on a soft surface, preferably a chair or bench. Kneel in front and lift the dumbbells toward your chest. Be sure your palms are facing up when you grip the weights.

A problem area for almost all people is the stomach. But a close second for many women can be the legs. Exercises for the stomach will be covered in Part 2 of this chapter. Here I will give some exercises for your upper and lower leg muscles. These leg exercises are a good supplement for any jogging program you might try.

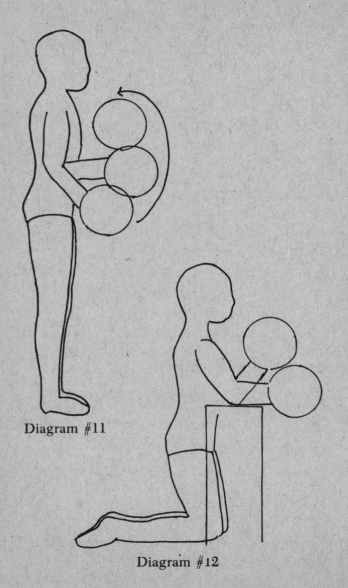

Diagram #11

Diagram #12

Exercise #6: *Half Squats* (See Diagram #13.)
Muscles: upper leg and thigh region

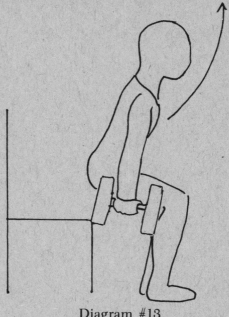

Diagram #13

Movement. Place a chair directly behind you.
Then hold dumbbells in each hand with your
arms straight down at your sides. Bend at your
knees to almost a sitting position, then return to
stand as before. Be careful not to sit on the chair;
and keep a steady rhythm.

Alternative exercise: *The Step-up* (See Diagrams
#14 & 15.) Muscles: thighs

Movement. Place a strong chair in front of you.
With a small dumbbell in each hand, step up

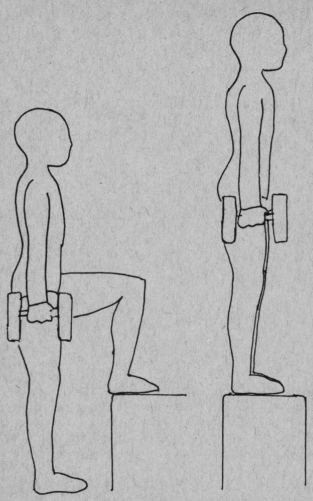

Diagrams #14 & 15

onto the seat of the chair. Use one leg and then the other to repeat the exercise.

Exercise #7: *Toe Raisers* (See Diagrams #16 & 17.) Muscles: lower legs (calves)

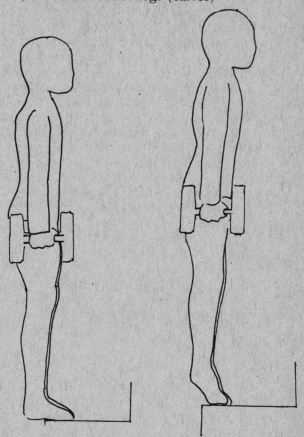

Diagrams #16 & 17

Movement. Stand straight gripping the dumbbells in each hand. Step up onto a stair or an object elevated a few inches off the ground.

Simply rise up to your tiptoes and then return to a flat-footed position only with heels overhanging the edge of the object. You should feel a burning sensation in your calf muscles after completing several repetitions. The burning sensation means you are doing the exercise properly.

Although dumbbell exercises may seem strange for women, they offer many dividends. The weights help to tighten loose and flabby skin quickly. And weight exercises properly done can improve posture, bust size and strength. The increased endurance and stamina will be apparent almost immediately in doing housework or away at the job. You will be sore after the first few workouts, but keep with the exercising because this only means that your muscles are getting proper exercise.

The following charted suggestions are given to help you get started on a weekly weight training program. On a three-day-a-week program, one day can emphasize the back and chest, one day the arms, and one day the legs. The stomach exercises which I will soon mention should be added, and in most cases they should be done on each exercise day.

DAY 1 CHEST, SHOULDERS AND UPPER BACK

No.	Exercise	Sets	Repetitions
1.	Standing flys	2	8-12
2.	Upright rowing	2	8-12
3.	Supine flys	2	8-12

DAY 2   ARMS

No.	Exercise	Sets	Repetitions
1.	Bent-arm pullovers	2	8-12
2.	Isolated curls	2	8-12
3.	Forward arm lift	2	8-12

DAY 3   LEGS

No.	Exercise	Sets	Repetitions
1.	Half squats	2	12-15
2.	Toe raisers	2-3	12-15
3.	Step-up	2	8-12

Part 2

General Exercises for Women

Just as I have done with the weighted exercises, I begin with the shoulders and work down to the calf muscles on the legs. I will give one basic exercise and then an alternative one. Two exercises for one muscle group will help to break the monotony of repetition in an exercise program.

You already may know exercises not mentioned in this part. If you know of a good exercise for a particular area, do it. Be careful to use only an exercise that you know to be effective. Also, do not eliminate exercises — only substitute.

When you substitute for an exercise make sure the new one attends to the same muscles that the old one attended to.

If you are just getting started, stick with the program examples discussed and charted at the end of this chapter. All of the suggested exercises are proven by use. Don't be timid or shy about exercise. Get right in and tackle these movements immediately.

Exercise #1: *Inclined Push-up*
(See Diagram #18.)
Muscles: shoulders, chest

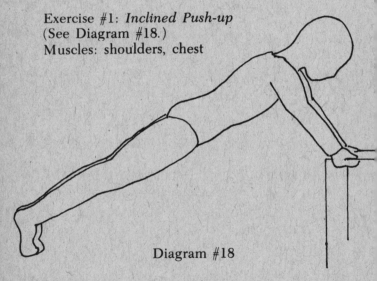

Diagram #18

Movement. Place a strong chair in front of you. Put your hands face down, palms on the far right and left hand sides of the seat. With your body straight and toes to the floor, lower your upper torso so that your chest touches the seat of the chair. Repeat. After a while try resting your hands on two chairs spaced the width of your shoulders. This will allow your chest to drop further down between the two chairs. You will feel some soreness when you first begin the push-up exercises.

Alternative exercise: *Conventional Push-up*
Muscles: shoulders, chest (See Diagram #19.)

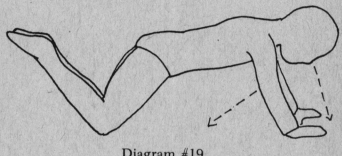

Diagram #19

Movement. Kneel on the floor and place palms down on the floor, shoulder width apart. Keep your back straight, bend at the elbows and touch your nose to the floor. The men's push-up requires that the legs be extended. But the women's push-up is done with the knees on the floor.

Exercise #2: *Arm Circles* (See Diagram #20.)
Muscles: arms and shoulders

Movement. Stand straight with your legs spread shoulder width apart. Extend your arms, elbows locked out to either side, then do small circles palms up. Start by doing several forward. Then reverse the direction.

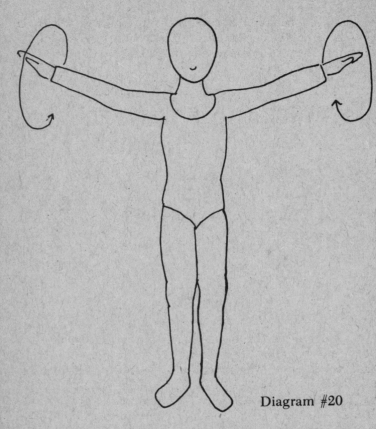

Diagram #20

Exercise #3: *Reverse Push-up* (See Diagram #21.)
Muscles: arms and chest

Movement. Follow the same procedures as done
with the conventional push-up. Only this time
face the fingers of both hands toward your body
instead of away from your body. Dip your torso
to the floor so that your chest just touches the
floor.

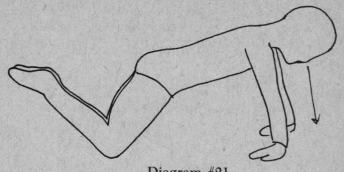

Diagram #21

Exercise #4: *Body Curl*
Muscles: lower back
(See Diagram #22.)

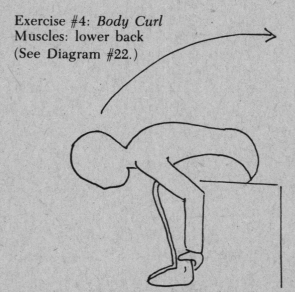

Diagram #22

Movement. Sit straight on a chair and then slowly reach down for your ankles and hold them for a
count of 5 seconds. Then return to an upright

posture. If your lower back muscles are giving you any trouble, begin this exercise by bending a little at a time until you can complete a full body curl.

Exercise #5: *Leg Raisers* (See Diagrams #23 & 24.) Muscles: lower back, abdomen

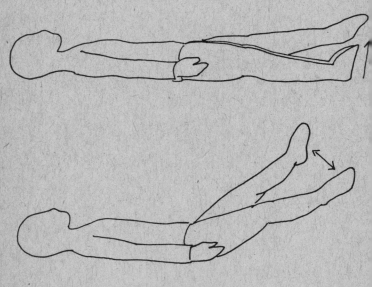

Diagrams #23 & 24

Movement. Lie flat on your back on the floor. Place your arms either at your side or clasp them behind your neck. On the count of one lift both legs together about 12 inches off the floor. On the count of two, spread your legs wide. On the third and fourth counts bring your legs together again and down.

Exercise #6: *Trunk Twist* (See Diagrams #25, 26, & 27.) Muscles: general back and waist

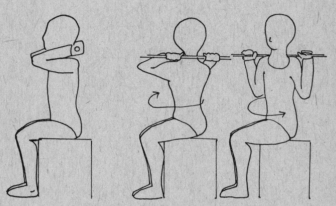

Diagrams #25, 26 & 27

Movement. Place a bar or a broom handle behind your neck and twist your torso and waist from side to side for 50–100 counts.

Alternative exercise: *Toe Touches* (See Diagrams #28 & 29.) Muscles: general back and waist

Movement. Stand straight, legs spread shoulder width and arms extended from your body. The first count of this four-count exercise is to touch your right hand to your left toe, keeping the same stance with your feet. Come up for the second count and reach for your right toes with your left hand for count three. Count four is up straight again. Try to complete 10 of these before jogging with your knees locked during the exercise.

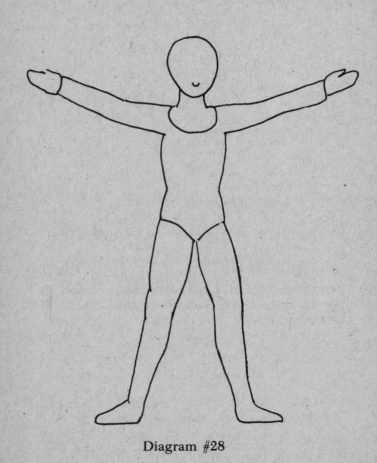

Diagram #28

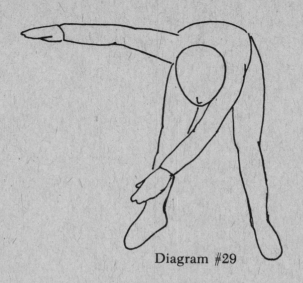

Diagram #29

Exercise #7: *Sit-ups* (See Diagrams #30 & 31.)
Muscles: stomach

Movement. Lie flat with your back to the floor.
Bend at the knees. Place hands on chest and sit
up until you reach your knees, then return. If
there is no one to hold your ankles, use the un-
derside of a bed. You can cushion your feet with
an old pillow.

Exercise #8: *Leg Extension* (See Diagram #32.)
Muscles: stomach

Movement. Lie flat on your back with legs extended. On the count of one, bring your knees
toward your chest. On the count of two, extend
them straight up. The counts of three and four
are a reverse of the above, bringing the legs back

115

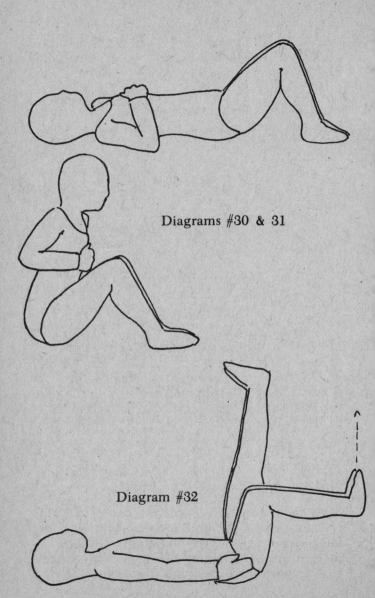

Diagrams #30 & 31

Diagram #32

to a curl position and then extending them to the ground. This is a beginning level exercise and can be supplemented by the leg raisers mentioned earlier.

Exercise #9: *Curl up*
Muscles: stomach
(See Diagram #33.)

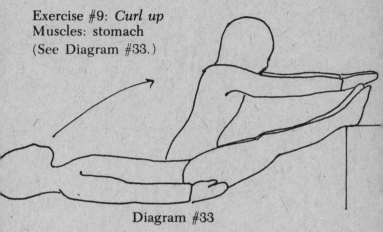

Diagram #33

Movement. Set your feet on a low chair. Lie with your back on the floor and sit up, reaching for your ankles. This is a difficult stomach exercise, so don't be discouraged if you cannot complete it right away. Work with the other abdominal exercises until the muscles are strong enough for this one.

Exercise #10: *Knee-bend* (See Diagram #34.)
Muscles: upper leg, thighs and hips

Movement. Stand with your arms outstretched in front of your body. Bend halfway down at your knees, keeping your arms straight in front of you. Be careful not to bend all the way down because a complete squat can injure the knees.

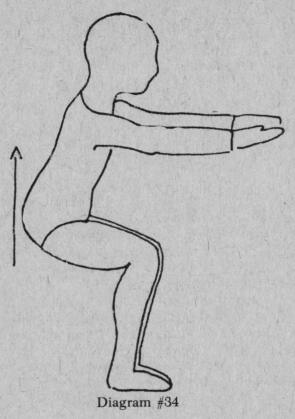

Diagram #34

The charts that follow have been designed to assist you in beginning your own exercise routine. I recommend that all physical fitness programs be supplemented by some jogging so that the heart muscle is exercised too. The three-day-a-week program can be used with these exercises. Note: the charts I provide divide the activities into three groups. First, the chest, upper back and shoulders are worked. Second, the arms

DAY 1 CHEST, SHOULDERS
AND UPPER BACK

No.	Exercise	Sets	Repetitions
1.	Jumping jack	1	20-25
2.	Push-up	2	8-12
3.	Arm circles	2	15-18/each arm
4.	Push-ups (inclined)	2	8-12
5.	Body curl	2	8-12

DAY 2 ARMS AND STOMACH

No.	Exercise	Sets	Repetitions
1.	Trunk twist	1	35-50
2.	Reverse push-up	2	8-12
3.	Leg raisers	2	6-12
4.	Arm circles	2	15-18/each arm
5.	Sit-ups	2	15-20

DAY 3 LEGS, STOMACH

No.	Exercise	Sets	Repetitions
1.	Toe touchers	1	12-15
2.	Leg extension & curl	2	8-12
3.	Knee-bend	2	12-15
4.	Toe raisers	2	12-15
5.	Leg raisers (side)	2	8-12/each leg

and the stomach, and finally the legs. The three-day-a-week program prevents 72 hours from elapsing before you work out again. You may do the work Monday, Wednesday, Friday or Tuesday, Thursday, Saturday. But it is important to set a regular schedule — same time, same place, same days each week. When setting your schedule keep in mind that it is best to work out one hour before or one hour after a meal. A workout before a meal is often good because exercise tends to *decrease* appetite for food.

The exercise chart on the preceding page will help get you started.

Alternative exercises can be substituted anywhere. If the number of repetitions is too much at first, do the best you can. If, on the other hand, you find yourself easily completing the repetitions, increase by one set per exercise: instead of doing two sets of an exercise, do three.

Now to answer some more of those questions you might be asking:

1. *When should I exercise?*

The answer is really anytime you can schedule it. The important word is "schedule." Find a time when you can do the workout three times a week. After work is as good a time as before work. And some people find that physical exercise relieves a great deal of the physical and emotional strain that goes with their daily work.

2. *What should I wear for exercise?*

Wear loose clothing that will not hinder circulation. Do not wear rubber clothing. Rubber suits hinder proper circulation and evaporation of sweat.

3. *Where should I exercise?*

These exercises are all designed for easy indoor

workouts. A carpet or some other form of padding should be on the floor to protect against injuries. If you want to exercise outdoors, grass is always a good surface.

4. *What footwear should be worn?*

Any rubberized tennis or athletic shoe will be fine for the exercises recommended in this chapter. If you want to combine these exercises with jogging or running, check Chapter 8 for advice on purchasing proper shoes.

5. *What about my difficulties with breathing when I do the exercises?*

Most of the troubles you will have with breathing arise from your poor physical condition. The more you do the exercises, therefore, the better your breathing will get.

But you may be troubled by improper breathing during exercise. For example, when doing push-ups you should breathe *out* while pushing up and *in* when coming down. When you exert the most you should be exhaling. Improper breathing inhibits circulation of the blood to the heart. Never hold your breath during exercises.

Start your exercise routine slowly. Don't get discouraged if you cannot complete all the suggested exercises with a high number of repetitions. Remember that Christian growth comes gradually and day by day. And as we walk with Christ through difficulties, we get stronger and stronger. What is required is the discipline *to keep going*. This is exactly what is required for physical fitness. Nearly all who quit do it in less than a week after they begin. So be encouraged and keep at the routine you establish.

Chapter Seven

Conditioning for Your Sport

"Total fitness implies the ability to function at an optimum level of efficiency in all daily living."
K.L. Jones

Some people find that they run out of energy in the second or third set of a tennis match. Others take that long awaited skiing weekend only to find that they spend most of the weekend in bed resting tired muscles.

If either one of these has been your problem, then this chapter might help you. To enjoy those trips to the mountains or evenings on the tennis court you must prepare for them. Listed in alphabetical order are popular recreational activities with suggestions for improving your performance and endurance.

Backpacking and Mountaineering

In the last decade mountain and wilderness travel has become very popular. Enthusiasts are braving the wildernesses of this nation and the world. And many who do not enjoy this great outdoor activity dislike it only because it requires too much physical stamina. But here are some suggestions that should assist you in preparation for time in the mountains and on the trails:

Cycling — high gear, 2–4 miles
Squats — 3 sets, 12–15 repetitions

Running bleachers or stairs — 100–200 steps
(count only the stairs going up)
Jogging — 2 or 3 miles
Mountain climbers — 3 sets, 10–15 repetitions

Basketball

Many people play weekend basketball games
at local schools or outdoors in parks or at home.
Even churches are responding to the popularity
of basketball and are including it in their list of
youth and adult activities. But basketball requires considerable endurance strength and
strong legs for jumping and rebounding. Try
these to help you:

Cycling — moderate gear, fast speed, 2–3 miles
Squats and toe raisers
Running bleachers or stairs — 100 to 200 stairs
(going up)
Wind sprints — 5x100 yds.
Jogging — 2 or 3 miles

Cycling

Cycling is rapidly becoming a popular
recreational activity in the U.S.A. And it is even
more popular in Europe. Cyclists decked out in
helmets, shorts, special shoes and even rear-view
mirror glasses are no longer an uncommon sight
on city streets.

Cycling is a physically demanding sport. The
primary muscles used are the thighs. Other
muscles involved include the calves, forearms
and the gluteal muscles. Some helpful exercises
include:

Jogging — 2 or 4 miles
Squats — 3 sets with 12–15 repetitions

Running bleachers or stairs — 125–200 stairs going up

Cycling is a good alternative to jogging if done vigorously. Depending on the speed at which you pedal, cycling can burn as many as 15 calories per minute.

Handball or Racquetball

Handball has been around for many years. The new craze for racquetball has swept the country only recently. Quick, short movements are required for both sports.

Quickness can be acquired through various exercises. A good one is the "shuttle run." Place two objects about 30 feet apart. The objects can be anything that you can easily carry, such as an eraser, a piece of wood or a glove. The shuttle run begins with the individual running as quickly as possible toward one of the objects, picking it up and carrying it back to the other one. Then pick up the other and carry it where the first one was sitting. By the time the shuttle has been completed you will have run about 40 yards. Keep doing the shuttle, leaving little time for rest between runs.

Diagram #1 Shuttle Run

Object	(30 feet)	Object

(Starting point)

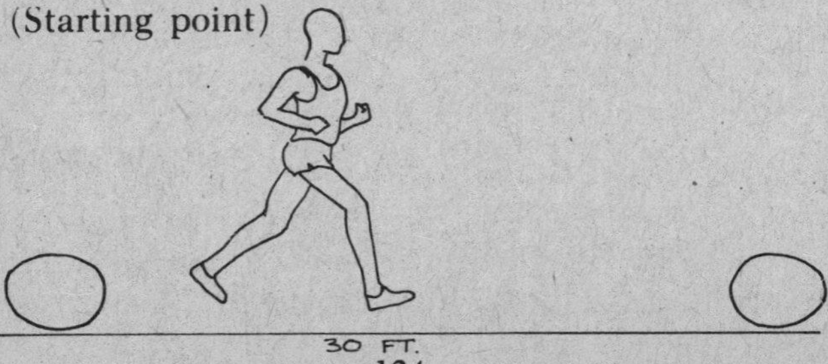

30 FT.

Since both racquetball and handball require leg strength and endurance, any leg exercise will be helpful.

Jogging — 2 to 3 miles
Sprints — 2 sprints of 10 yds., 2 sprints of 20 yds., 2 sprints of 30 yds.
Squats — 2 sets with 15–18 repetitions
Mountain climbers — 3 sets of 12–15 repetitions
Running bleachers or stairs — 75–150 steps up

Marathon Running

Experienced joggers and runners who yearn for the pain of a marathon may follow the workout schedule to prepare for the 26 mile 385-yard race. A marathon run is a tremendous strain on the entire body. Training requires months, even if you have been running regularly.

Here is a running program that will prepare you for a marathon race.

Day	Workout	Mileage	Benefit
Monday	1x8-12 miles	8-12 miles	endurance
Tuesday	2x5 miles	10 miles	endurance
Wednesday	3x3 miles	9 miles	endurance-pace
Thursday	4x2 miles	8 miles	pace-speed
Friday	5x1 miles	5 miles	pace-speed
Saturday	1x8-12 miles	8-12 miles	endurance
Sunday	none	none	rest

Your weekly total of miles should be between 45 and 60. The more miles you can do a week the better your chances of finishing well. You should do a long run on Saturday. The pace of the long run can be fairly slow, but don't stop.

If the 45 to 60 mile program is too difficult for you, begin with less distance a week and work your way up to it. Before you enter a marathon you should be able to do a 15-mile run without too much discomfort. An important training aid is the daily running diary where you keep track of distance, time, route and pesty dogs.

A major problem for any distance runner is the dog that suddenly appears and wants to fight. A loud shout will often stop a dog in his tracks (it's the noise that does it, so shout as loudly as you can). Sticks and stones are good armament as well. But if the dog is trained to attack, all you can do is try to defend yourself. Keep your head down and your body as low as possible to the ground. Don't expect much help from the dog's owner (he or she usually isn't any smarter than the dog, and will likely accuse you of attacking the dog!). But take the owner's name and address. Even if you don't report him to the proper authorities, he will think that you will and he may decide to chain his dog.

Alpine Skiing

In most areas of the U.S.A. skiing is a one-season sport. When the season arrives, therefore, most ski enthusiasts are woefully unprepared for the rigors of the sport. But you can prepare yourself. The legs are the most critical area to prepare. During a downhill run, the body must remain in nearly a seated position with all of the weight thrown on the thighs and knees. (See Diagram #2.)

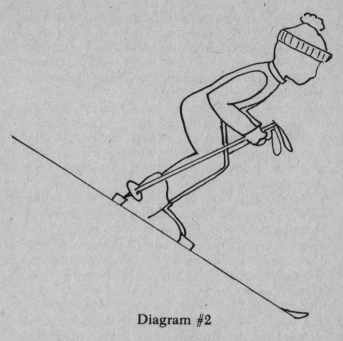

Diagram #2

Incorporate some or all of the suggestions below and you will be ready when the snow begins to fall.

Cycling — 2 or 3 miles, three days a week
Running up bleachers or stairs — 75 to 100 steps
Mountain climbers — 2 sets with 8–12 repetitions
Squats — 2 sets with 12–15 repetitions

Swimming

Although most people swim only for pleasure, swimming can be one of the best forms of exercise if done in a disciplined way. But swimming has so many variations of strokes that it is difficult to give specific exercises to improve performance. Since so many muscles are used in swimming, any and all of the endurance exercises recommended in this book will help. Highly recommended are jogging, push-ups, sit-ups and squats.

Tennis

Another very popular game of recent years is tennis. Today new homes are being built with courts on the properties or with special access to a local court.

Tennis is a good sport because it does not require a great deal of strength. Yet like handball and racquetball it is a quick game and requires many moves. Generally tennis players find that their weakest muscles are in their wrists. But the wrist can be greatly improved by the wrist curl exercise noted earlier.

Endurance is also an important factor for tennis. Improving your endurance will improve your game. And daily jogging or cycling is probably the best way to improve endurance.

Some activities have not been mentioned in this chapter simply because they do not really provide that much beneficial activity for the human body. These activities include golf, bowling, archery and sailing. The chart below lists sport activities and their rank in terms of effectiveness for conditioning the body for health.

If you are not presently enjoying some regular recreational activity such as the ones mentioned in this chapter, it would be good for you to adopt one. But start doing one that promotes cardiovascular fitness. Such an activity will be of the greatest benefit to you. Be careful not to substitute a game like tennis for your regular fitness workouts. You need to do both. Tennis itself is not sufficient as a means to work all the muscles.

Rating	Activity	Muscle Groups	Effectiveness
1.	Running	Legs, buttocks	heart & lungs, leg tone
2.	Cycling	Legs, forearms	heart & lungs, leg tone
3.	Swimming	Legs, arms (chest)	heart & lungs, muscle tone
4.	Backpacking	Legs, buttocks, back, shoulders	heart & lungs, leg tone
5.	Racquet and Handball	Legs, buttocks	some heart & lungs, leg tone
6.	Skiing x-country	Legs, buttocks	heart & lungs, leg tone
7.	Ice Skating	Legs, buttocks	some heart & lungs, leg tone
8.	Skiing Alpine	Legs	little heart & lungs
9.	Tennis	Legs	little heart & lungs, some leg tone
10.	Badminton	Legs	little heart & lungs

Chapter Eight

Fitness Equipment

The fitness industry has capitalized on the recent craze for better health. Today, there are more varieties of shoes, weights and body building kits than ever before. Stores have expanded their sporting goods departments to include the many new innovations now available. Magazine ads boast enormous results "in just 60 seconds a day," and health spas are offering "once a year specials" that last all year. This chapter is devoted to those who wish to expand their fitness workouts by setting up their own "mini gyms." It will also include shoes and jogging paraphernalia. The prices quoted are the mean retail costs of various articles and may vary in different stores and towns.

Weights

Weights come in three basic forms: 1) Standard iron, 2) Standard plastic coated, and 3) Olympic. The Olympic weight sets are not recommended unless you can bench press 225 pounds or more. The standard iron sets usually come with collars, bars and weights. The iron weights are the most durable. Plastic coated concrete weights eventually crack with time and weathering. And once the casings crack you should get rid of them because they can break apart.

Weight Type	Total Weight	Mean Cost	Weight Increments
Iron Standard	110 lbs.	$40-50	2½, 5, 10, 25, 50
Plastic Standard	110 lbs.	$30-35	2½, 5, 10, 25
Olympic	300-320 lbs.	$325-400	2½, 5, 10, 25, 35, 45

The Olympic weight sets must be used only with heavier benches designed for the heavier weights. Also the width of the bar on an Olympic set requires a considerable amount of room in the workout area since it extends over 7 feet.

Benches

Weight benches are usually easy to find and generally not too expensive. The most important thing to look for in a weight bench is its sturdiness. Price is generally a good indicator of the quality of the weight bench. There are varieties of benches: some are made with leg units built into them. Other benches have adjustable backs for doing the incline bench press and isolated curls. A good bench will generally cost between $40 and $100. Beware of benches that cost less. The cheaper benches will not hold much weight safely. Be sure to check to see that the bench is assembled properly before you use it.

Exercycles

One commonly bought and rarely used piece of equipment is the exercycle. The exercycle is a simple fitness product that enables one to ride in-

Accessories

Item	Purpose	Cost
Lifting belt	back support	$25
Curling bar	bicep and tricep isolation	$15
Sit up boards	sit ups and stomach	$20
Ankle weights	worn while jogging or walking	$10
Hand grips	forearms and wrists	$4-5
Jump rope	builds legs, stamina	$5
Pull up bar	back, arms and shoulders	$8
Trim twister	stomach and sides	$10 up

doors. This is especially useful in parts of the country where the weather is poor. The various options add or subtract from the price of the exercycle. Most options include speedometers, tension adjustments, rotating handlebars or seats, and timer. The only necessary option is the tension adjustment, and most cycles have knobs already built in. This enables you to improve by making the pedaling more difficult or loosen the tension and pedal more freely. A watch or clock will tell you how long you have pedaled, eliminating the necessity for a timer or speedometer. An exercycle can be purchased from $40.00 and up, but be sure it is sturdy and *most* important, use it! The exercycle is a good warm-up exercise and is definitely a good investment.

Shoes

The most important single piece of equipment you can buy for your body is a pair of shoes. There are many styles of running and jogging shoes on the market. Unfortunately many of the shoes bought and sold today are simply cheap copies of the best shoes.

When buying footwear it is important to recognize that tennis, basketball and jogging require different shoes. A shoe is designed for a particular activity on a particular surface. A tennis shoe is designed for quick stopping and starting and must have the strength for lateral movement. Jogging shoes must have a certain degree of roundness on the heels and toes to help provide a fluid motion while running. If you attempt to run in a tennis or basketball shoe, you will discover that your foot slaps the ground in an awkward way. You will then adjust your running style to the shoe and begin to run improperly, and you may injure yourself if you continue to run. Likewise, playing tennis in a jogging shoe increases your chances of injury because the jogging shoe lacks the support necessary for tennis.

The surface you play on is also an important consideration. The jogger must have an idea of the surface he will most likely be jogging on, whether it be asphalt, concrete, grass, tarton or gravel. The handball, racquetball, tennis and basketball player must also know if they will be playing indoors or outdoors.

The three basic soles for jogging and running shoes are these: 1) waffle, 2) riveted, 3) flat or slightly grooved. The waffle soles have bumps that protrude from the bottom of the shoe like tiny rubber spikes. One advantage of the waffle bottoms is that they provide some additional cushioning. A disadvantage is that the waffle soles wear more quickly in some areas than in others, and the ankles then may twist as the foot lands. Injury can follow. The ridged or sawtooth soles are good for cross country and hill jogging but tend to be too hard for asphalt and concrete surfaces.

The flat soled jogging shoes function best on flat surfaces, e.g., tracks, streets, etc. The flat soled shoes are not good for jogging on hills or cross-country courses because they provide little traction.

The upper portion of the jogging and running shoe is also varied. Today's shoes are most commonly covered with a nylon upper, which is reinforced with leather in stress areas, i.e., toe, heel and arch. Nylon is light and flexible, allowing the shoes to "break in" easier. The older leather shoes are rarely used except on rough terrain. A more recent development is the use of "Mesh Nylon" a criss-cross netlike material that allows the feet to breathe easier.

For the beginning jogger a flat soled shoe with a nylon upper should suffice. Be sure to purchase name brands, this will usually assure that you'll get a quality shoe. "Adidas" has the largest line of athletic footwear; however, Puma, Tiger and Nike are also reliable shoes. Don't hesitate to pay a few dollars more for name brands. In the long run (no pun intended) they will fit better, give better support and help prevent needless injury. Good jogging or running shoes will generally cost between $25—40. It is also safest to purchase from an independently owned sporting goods store or athletic specialists. Beware of regular shoe stores which sometimes substitute good-looking nylon shoes for the real things. The independently run stores will in some cases resole your old shoes.

Keep an eye on the inside cushion of any athletic footwear. The cushioning helps to protect you from those aggravating injuries that come from constantly striking your feet on a hard surface. A new type of inner cushioning called Spenco is now on the market and is very useful for protecting the feet while running on hard surfaces. Lastly be sure your shoes have a firm heel counter to help protect against heel injuries. Shoes also must be soft and flexible, especially under the ball of the foot. A flexible shoe will enable the feet to roll with your stride.

Stop Watches

For those joggers and runners who are serious about running, some type of timing piece is a necessity. If you jog alone a stop watch can be that imaginary runner beside you prodding you on. A watch allows you to pace yourself over short or long distances (see pace chart in Chapter 5). An ordinary metal cased stop watch is generally durable and accurate and costs between $25—40. A shoe string tied to the top of the watch enables you to have a better hold on the watch while running. Wrap the string through the metal loop and then tie a strong knot in it; while jogging or running wrap the string around your wrist.

Digital stop watches are now available in both hand-held and wrist models. Digital watches are accurate, easy to read and light weight. Prices for digital watches start at about $30.

Warm-up Suits

Warm-up and sweat-type suits are vital in parts of the country where temperatures are cool and cold. Generally a warm-up garment should be worn when your body chills. This will vary between individuals, and women more than men will chill faster. If you are a heavy "sweater," your chances of catching a cold increase as the cool air comes into contact with the perspiration on the exposed skin. Muscles are also pulled more often in cold temperatures. Your muscles act in much the same way that a rubber band does, stretching easily in warm and humid weather and becoming stiff and brittle when cold. Some important factors to consider before purchasing sweat suits are:

Be sure the garment fits loose enough in order to allow your body room to move while exercising. The body's ability to breathe is also hampered by rubbers and plastics, both of which should never be worn while exercising. Plastics and rubbers inhibit proper evaporation of perspiration. The best-looking tennis attire is tight-fitting and most impractical for exercising. The best warm-ups are the not-so-sporty, baggy sweats which cost around $15. The tennis suits can cost as much as five or six times more. The baggier warm-ups come in four basic colors: grey, red, navy and green. A wool cap is a very good investment if you run in cool or cold weather. Most of the body heat escapes through the head. A $3 wool cap will keep that heat in and top off your outfit too.

Additional information about purchasing footwear may be obtained by writing

All Pro Sporting Goods
16919 Ventura Bl.
Encino, CA 91316.

Chapter Nine

Attitudes

The Attitudes of Others

Although you may wish to improve the condition of your body, you will soon discover that there are many people who are simply uninterested in exercise. But there seems to be many more who are distinctly hostile, and the heckling you may have to endure can be a trial.

Keep in mind, however, that in most cases opposition to your exercise routine is often rooted in both jealousy and guilt. They know that you are doing something good to yourself. They feel they should be doing it too. But they don't want to take the initial steps. So be kind, patient and encouraging toward them. Their stock remark will be a quotation from the Bible: "Bodily exercise profiteth little . . ." Your response should be that it "profiteth" much more than a diet of cookies, cake and potato chips.

Your Own Attitude

It is important that you not be diverted from your exercise program. But it is equally important that you not have the "I'm better than you" attitude. Rather, be unobtrusive in your exercise program. If the hostility comes from your own family, try to find a time to exercise that will not inconvenience them. Above all, don't let your exercise program get in the way of your obligations to your family. And be sure not to push your exercise program upon others. You can certainly recommend it to others (even as you recommend your relationship with Christ to others.

The worst opposition you will face is your own self. The human mind is most creative when thinking of reasons not to exercise. But next to laziness, discouragement is also a problem. Have you ever shared Christ with an unbeliever, only to receive the answer back: "Oh, I've tried Christianity and it didn't work for me?" But you don't *try* exercising, you *do* exercises. And you don't *try* Christianity, you *live* Christianity. To discipline ourself toward a new pattern of life will be difficult: It will be especially difficult if you have never regularly exercised before.

Remind yourself of the benefits you receive from exercise. Expect the program to be somewhat difficult at first. Remember that anything worth doing is difficult to do. Remember also that 54% of all Americans die from cardiovascular diseases, such as heart attack, stroke, and hardening of the arteries. Exercise prevents such diseases.

In fact there is *no* reason why you need to *ever* suffer from heart disease, providing you take the proper measures to prevent it. The human body's 60,000 blood vessels nourish its 300,000,000,000,-000 cells! You would need to travel from the East coast to the West coast 20 times to reach the distance covered by the blood vessels within this intricate mechanism called the body. The tiny heart weighs less than a pound, yet pumps 1,-000,000 gallons of blood each year. That's the equivalent to filling nearly 44 swimming pools! You can never flip a switch to let your heart rest; as long as you live your heart will be pumping about 100,000 times every day. You are the *only* one that can keep this most important muscle functioning as it should, no one can do it for you and the older you become the more critical it becomes to take care of.

If you are past middle age, don't waste precious time *thinking* about exercising. Start doing it! For those who are young, there is no better time to start on a fitness program than *now*. Start slowly. But be consistent.

Parents should not discourage their children from participating in an exercise program. If you jog, you can let your children ride along on a bicycle or jog beside you. This builds a good foundation for their futures. The sooner a child begins physical activities the easier it will be for that child to discipline himself for a lifetime program. So, parents, be good examples to your children.

The purpose of this book has been both to open your eyes to the dangers of not maintaining a physical fitness program and to show the benefits of keeping the temple of God healthy. Although we do not carry our physical bodies into eternity, physical fitness will prolong our usefulness and enhance our work for the kingdom. But never substitute exercise for time spent on the essentials of knowing God. Just as there is no substitute for bodily fitness, there is no substitute for time with the creator. "Delight yourself in the Lord; and He will give you the desires of your heart" (Psalms 37:4).

GLOSSARY

Barbell. A long narrow bar which is usually iron extending approximately six feet and designed to be used with both hands.

Burn-out. A slang term used to describe the exhaustedness of the muscles when they can lift no more weight.

Calorie. Measurement of heat energy.

Cardiovascular. Involving the heart and blood vessels.

Dumbbell. Small bar, usually iron about 12 to 18 inches in length and designed to be used with one hand.

Exhausting the Muscles. Continuous use of the muscle until you can complete no more repetitions.

Jog. To move at a slow monotonous pace.

Lap. One full time around a regulation size oval track, 440 yards or 400 meters.

Max. Short for maximum. The greatest amount of weight an individual can lift at a particular exercise.

Pace. The ability to maintain a consistent speed while jogging or running.

Pulse Rate, or PR, is the number of beats per minute the heart is pumping.

Repetition. The number of times an exercise is completed within a set.

Run. Faster than a jog and slower than a sprint.

Set. The number of times a particular exercise is done, i.e. bench press; 3 sets of 8 repetitions.

Sprint. A quick short run.

Squat. Lifting by bending at the knees to a seated position.

Tone. The outward appearance of a muscle or muscles.

Valsalva Effect, or Valsalva maneuver, is the process of making a forceful attempt at exhaling while keeping the nostrils and mouth shut.

Warm-up. Preliminary stretching and preparation of muscles for exercising.

BIBLIOGRAPHY

The West Point Fitness and Diet Book,
Col. James L. Anderson and Martin Cohen, 1977.

The Lazy Man's Guide to Physical Fitness,
Kenneth D. Rose with Jack Dies Martin, 1974.

Spiritual and Physical Health,
Charles S. Price, 1936.

Thinking Life Through,
Connors, 1970.

The Human Body,
Martin Keen, 1961.

Basic Nutrition and Diet Therapy,
Corinne H. Robinson, 3rd Ed.

BFCO Handbook on Body Building,
  Dimensions III
Jones, Shainberg, Byer, 1976.

Special thanks to Winston Severn of "ALL PRO" Sporting Goods.

Scriptural Sources (no symbols used):
The *New American Standard Bible,* Copyright by the Lockman Foundation, 1971; the *King James Version;* and the *Scofield Reference Bible,* Copyright renewed 1937, 1945 by Oxford University Press.